MY LAST DEGREE:

A Therapist Goes Home After a Stroke

REBECCA DUTTON

DISCLAIMER

This book is not a substitute for formal rehabilitation services that individualize treatment for your specific needs. Nor is it a comprehensive review of the literature that describes every problem associated with every kind of stroke. This is the story of one person's stroke experience that attempts to make stroke survivors and their families better consumers of rehabilitation and community services. When readers understand how a stroke can affect home life, it is easier to share specific concerns with the rehabilitation team. Each topic includes suggestions readers should consider, but these suggestions are not an exhaustive list that covers all the issues that can affect your situation. Suggestions illustrate the active role that consumers can take to maximize their recovery.

Acknowledgments

It took a small army to get me ready to live in my own home after a stroke. The way each person helped me are described in the book. I'd especially like to thank Arlene for taking me into her home for three months and Janet for editing this book. I'd like to thank my brothers Mark and Jim and my friends Ann, Anne, Bobbie, Greg, Joanne, John, Karen, Mike, Mirah, Patti, Peggy, Raffaela, and Suzanne. I'd like to thank Dr. Terry, my brace man Wayne, and my therapists Carrie, David, Doug, Kathy, Kim, Leslie, Lincoln, Melissa, Michelle, and Tracy.

Several people helped me field-test the Test of Bilateral Hand Use (TEBHU). I'd like to thank the eleven stroke survivors who volunteered to take the TEBHU. I'd like to thank Melissa and John at St. Lawrence Rehabilitation Center in Lawrenceville, NJ. I'd like to thank Shelly and Nancy at JFK Johnson Rehabilitation Institute in Edison, NJ. I'd like to thank the following graduate students in Occupational Therapy at Kean University in Union, NJ: Brooke, Erika, Jamie, and Khara.

TABLE OF CONTENTS

CHAPTER 1: INTRODUCTION 1
My Two Strokes 1
How Hard is It? 4
Keeping Hope Alive 6
Saving My Sanity on the Weekends 7
Dealing with the Hospital System 8
Setting the Stage for Success 9
The Bottom Line 10

CHAPTER 2: REGAINING MOBILITY 13
Bed Mobility is a Burden 13
Standing Up and Going Floppo 15
Wheelchairs Can Wreck a Home 17
Squats are Your Friend 18
Balance Skills You Need at Home 21
Canes, Walkers, Braces, and Shoes 23
Multitasking Means Having a Life 25
The Most Dangerous Room is the Kitchen 27
Inexpensive Home Modifications Prevent Falls 28
Low Endurance is a Deal Breaker 30
The Bottom Line 32

CHAPTER 3: RECOVERY OF AN ARM AND A HAND 34
The Functional Value of the Hemiplegic Arm 34
Why Recovery is Harder for the Hand 38
Good News from Constraint-Induced Therapy 39
Electrical Stimulation for the Hemiplegic Hand 40
Evaluation of the Hemiplegic Hand is Outdated 42
Making the Hemiplegic Hand Functional 44
Finding the Ceiling 52
The Bottom Line 54

CHAPTER 4: BASIC SELF-CARE 58
Gadgets versus What You Carry with You 58
Getting Clean Sitting on a Shower Chair 60

You Can Floss One-Handed 64
Does Leaning Over Help You Don a Shirt? 65
Donning a Short-Leg Brace the Easy Way 66
Having the Energy to Worry about Your Hair...................68
Elastic Shoelaces Come in What Colors?.........................69
Don't Forget Outerwear...75
Houdini Puts on a Bra One-Handed..................................78
The Bottom Line 80

CHAPTER 5: ADVANCED ADLs IN THE HOME 81
A Small Army Got Me into My New Home......................82
Baby Steps Come First..83
Mom, Answer the Phone..84
Taking Meds Wrong Can Kill You....................................85
Transporting Objects without Taking All Day 87
Bill Collectors Don't Care If You Have a Stroke.............88
A Computer isn't a Luxury 90
I'm Not Washing My Clothes at a Laundromat.................92
A Microwave Oven Saves the Day 94
Food Prep with Low and High Tech Solutions.................95
Cleaning Varies from Easy to Difficult 99
Small Tasks that Fall through the Cracks 103
The Bottom Line 104

CHAPTER 6: ADVANCED ADLs IN THE COMMUNITY 106
Keys, Money, and Purses Come First..............................106
Eating Out Takes Practice...107
Paratransit Really Works 109
Shopping with Paratransit...112
Shopping for Clothes is Like Going to War 115
Good Timing is Free 116
Maneuvering in Crowds that Sit Down 117
Americans Love to Drive...119
Showering While I'm On the Road Again.......................126
A Plane Sounds Better than an MRI 127
Returning to Work 130
The Bottom Line..132

CHAPTER 7: PAIN CAN RUIN EVERYTHING 134
A Subluxed Shoulder Really Hurts 134
Vigilance Fixes a Swollen Hand 135
A Cold Foot Can Ruin Your Sleep 136
Do Shoulder Range of Motion Lying Down 136
How Do You Relax Tight, Painful Muscles? 137
The Bottom Line 141

CHAPTER 8: RECOVERY OF A PERSON 142
Choosing to Live 142
Regaining a Social Life 143
My Perfectionism Comes Back to Bite Me 146
Stress Management Gets Out of the Back Seat 148
Being Depressed for Hours Instead of Months 149
Love and Lust 151
A Stroke Teaches You Want versus Need 154
The Big Question I Asked Myself 155

Appendix A: Assisted Living 159

Appendix B: Concierge Service Anyone? 169

Appendix C: Council on Independent Living 171

Index 173

About the Author 175

CHAPTER 1

INTRODUCTION

As a baby boomer, I used to feel a vague sense of anxiety about the aging of America. Adults age sixty-five and older are going to make up twenty percent of the U.S. population by 2030 – but that feels so far away. Besides, as an occupational therapist (OT), I was going to help baby boomers "age in place," which means staying in your own home as you get older. This feel-good philosophy didn't become personal until I had a stroke at age fifty-eight. How was I going to live in a house with one bathroom on the second floor when I couldn't even walk up one step? Still, I had an option my grandparents didn't have. I could go to an assisted-living facility.

Middle-class families are going to suffer sticker shock when they look into assisted living. Here is an example of what one assisted-living facility costs. A *studio* apartment, three meals a day, and amenities like daily activities, cost $3,000 a month or $36,000 a year in 2004. In 2008 it cost $3,500 a month or $42,000 a year. If you actually need assistance in an assisted-living facility, that costs extra. These facility-based expenses don't cover health insurance, medicine, the clothes on your back, or toilet paper. I've never been poor, but the money I set aside for retirement will last only a few years with this kind of financial drain. Since I had a stroke at fifty-eight, my only long-term financial option was to return home and stay as long as possible. It took a miracle and a small army to help me get there.

My Two Strokes

Spring break was over and I was looking forward to teaching my favorite module on stroke rehabilitation. While getting ready for work, I couldn't stop falling backwards on the bed as I closed one eye to put on eye make-up. As a therapist, I knew this wasn't normal. I could still walk with both eyes open so I foolishly drove myself to the hospital. I walked into the emergency room and signed myself in. A few hours later, a neurologist came to see me and confirmed my worst fear. I was having a stroke. By dinnertime I was paralyzed.

My stroke was caused by cholesterol building up inside the small blood vessels of my brain. This is called chronic small blood vessel disease. Cholesterol build-up narrows the blood vessels and increases blood pressure, just as you increase water pressure by partially covering the end of a garden hose with your thumb. Increased blood pressure can make tiny blood vessels burst and disrupt blood flow to the brain. The episodes of sudden dizziness I experienced over the years made sense when I saw my MRI with numerous pinpoints of light shining through the sub-cortical areas of my brain. These tiny areas of brain damage don't have a permanent effect at first, but when enough pinholes get close to each other they collapse into a lake and produce a lacunar stroke (lacunar means lake). My "lake" formed in a structure called the pons, which is the bridge to the cerebellum. This was good news because a stroke that cuts off the blood supply to the cerebellum doesn't produce the severe cognitive and language deficits associated with other types of stroke. The bad news is that this stroke made my right arm and leg flaccid and severely impaired my balance. My right side is still partially paralyzed so I refer to it as my hemiplegic side.

Small blood vessel disease is frustrating because surgery can't save you. Surgery works only for *large* blood vessel disease, like inserting a stent in an artery after a balloon flattens the cholesterol build-up. I tried for years to get my high cholesterol down because heart disease runs in my family. Statin drugs made my triglycerides go sky high. Triglycerides are another group of fatty acids in the blood that are associated with heart disease. Statin drugs also gave me severe constipation that was relieved only by taking an increasing number of laxative pills. I tried six statin drugs before I found one I could tolerate with the help of Miralax powder, which pulls water into the gut. I don't know how long my blood pressure was intermittently high. It would be high one day and normal when I went back the next day, so my internist didn't prescribe blood pressure medicine. After six years, I decided to see a cardiologist. She started me on blood pressure medicine and prescription-strength fish oil to lower my triglycerides, but it was too late. The damage was already done. Tell the people you love not to ignore high cholesterol or high blood pressure because they don't feel sick.

With nothing to do but lie in bed in the Intensive Care Unit, I tried to touch my left index finger to my nose but kept missing. In addition to paralysis on my right side, my left side was also affected. When I told the neurologist about this, he ordered another MRI. The MRI showed narrowing of the basilar artery that supplies blood to the cerebellum.

The cerebellum controls coordination as well as balance. I had strength in what people called my "sound arm," but lost fine-motor control of this arm. I had to wear a bib for weeks because I couldn't get a utensil to my mouth without spilling food on my shirt. When I pulled my shoe off, it went flying across the room. When I reached for a glass, I knocked it over because I couldn't stop my arm as it got close to the glass. I lost track of how many times I spilled while trying to pour myself a glass of water. The glass always overflowed because my hand couldn't pull the pitcher back in time. When I tried to click on a computer icon, my hand pushed the mouse well past the mark.

These uncontrolled movements were infuriating because I couldn't stop them even though I knew they were going to happen. They were like the super-fast movements that pull your hand away from a hot stove before you have time to form a conscious thought to move. Incoordination can be a confusing deficit. People who saw me walk with a cane in my left hand didn't know I had trouble controlling a spoon with this hand. This deficit made me hysterical. How could I go home with poor coordination in one hand and paralysis in the other?

Theories of motor control don't have many suggestions for treating incoordination so I learned what worked by trial and error. When I reached for an object, I had better control if I moved slowly. It helped to imagine that I was reaching for an object embedded in Jell-O. When my left hand fumbled with an object, it helped to stop and rest for a few seconds. When I got back to the task I was struggling with, I was always more coordinated. This left-sided incoordination gradually went away, so I refer to my left side as my sound side.

Incoordination affected the oral muscles so my speech was slurred and difficult to understand at first. Incoordination of my diaphragm was an even bigger problem. At first, I exhaled explosively with one big gasp. I had to take an extra breath to finish even one sentence. Now I can sustain a longer exhalation, which means I can say more before running out of breath. This gives me the option of choosing natural places in a sentence to take an extra breath to make my meaning more apparent. I speak clearly enough for people to understand me on the telephone, but I slur my words when I get tired at night. It's still tiring to project my voice for extended periods of time in a group because I have to take deep breaths to make my voice heard.

A scary fact about incoordination and poor balance is that people ignore them as warning signs of stroke because they are rarely mentioned in public service announcements. I had another small stroke two years later and had to go back to rehab to learn how to walk again. Yet even a neurologist suggested that my sudden return of impaired balance was probably caused by an ear infection. It wasn't until I told him I had acquired double vision and lost the ability to distinguish between hot and cold in my hemiplegic leg that he agreed I had another stroke. The American Stroke Association (2007) estimates that twenty-five percent of strokes cut off the blood supply to the back of the brain where balance, coordination, and vision are controlled. A sudden onset of impaired balance, coordination, or vision should be taken as seriously as impaired speech or paralysis of a limb.

How Hard is It?

Movie and TV scripts create unrealistic fantasies about how people recover from a physical disability. Stroke survivors need a story of recovery that is both hopeful and realistic. Regaining control of my body was harder than I ever imagined. In the beginning, when a therapist asked me to lift my hemiplegic leg, it was like asking me to lift a car. Well, maybe not a car, but my hemiplegic leg felt as though it weighed a hundred pounds. Moving my hemiplegic arm and leg took more concentration than learning how to drive a stick-shift car. Rehabilitation is mentally as well as physically exhausting.

One way to describe how difficult it is to move a paralyzed limb is to tell you what an experienced skier told me when he explained how to turn while skiing downhill. To turn, you shift seventy-five percent of

4

your weight onto the inside edge of the downhill ski. These directions don't mean much to a non-skier. I felt the same way when my therapists asked me to make a fist or take a step. I didn't have a clue about how to follow my therapists' commands. In the first month after my stroke, I performed simple movements only by concentrating as hard as I have ever concentrated in my entire life and repeating every motion dozens of times.

As you do a movement over and over again, the brain grows new branches around the damaged area. These new branches are called collateral sprouting. Collateral sprouting is tricky because being able to grow new connections doesn't mean you can find them. I had a wonderful physical therapist (PT) who waited four to five seconds after she gave me a command so I had time to figure out how to do what she wanted. I never lost the ability to feel where my limbs were in space when someone else moved them, but I had a terrible time figuring out how to control the muscles I wanted to use. Those extra seconds Michelle gave me allowed me to search for the new connections my brain had created so I could do the movements she had asked for.

I never appreciated how difficult breathing can be for someone with a stroke. As a therapist, I had told my clients to stop holding their breath because it increases blood pressure. To my horror, I repeatedly held my breath when I was straining. Awareness and good intentions were not enough. I didn't learn how to breathe properly until six months after my stroke when a PT in outpatient rehab had me lean against a closed door and breathe in when I slid down and breathe out when I slid up. Now I know that if a movement makes me strain, I have to stop and plan when to breathe *before* I start to move again. This gives me one more thing I have to control in addition to my hemiplegic limbs. However, keeping my blood pressure down is important, so I try to breathe properly when I'm straining.

Finally, stroke rehabilitation is hard because it never completely ends. After being treated by three inpatient therapists, two home health therapists, and two outpatient therapists, I had been assigned dozens and dozens of home exercises. There was no way I was going to do all those exercises. Therapists call this "non-compliance" because each therapist sees only what he or she thinks the client should do. Xerox machines make it easy for therapists to overwhelm clients with home programs.

When I went through the therapy process again after a second stroke, I asked my therapists to help me prioritize. I made a list of exercises I had been given by previous therapists that I was still doing. I showed the list to my new set of therapists and asked them which ones they thought were important to keep doing. When my new therapists wanted to add their own exercises, I made them aware of my current total. When the total got too high, I asked each therapist which two or three of their exercises they felt most strongly about. I can't maintain my commitment to a home program when it cuts into my time for socializing and having fun.

Keeping Hope Alive

In the beginning, being a therapist was a hindrance. For the first month, I scared myself half to death by picturing everything that could go wrong. My fear made me intermittently hysterical and disrupted my early treatment. I tried not to think about what life would be like with strokes on both sides, but sometimes the dam burst and I sobbed for several minutes.

I don't know how I would have coped with these **emotional meltdowns** without the compassion of therapists and friends. When I sobbed uncontrollably, my PT would roll my wheelchair to an empty corner of the gym, squat down to look me in the eye, and talk to me. It didn't matter what Michelle was saying. She distracted me and made me feel less alone. She had me go back to work when I calmed down, which gave me something to think about besides my fear. A friend used another approach when she came to visit and found me crying in my room. Bobbie put her arm around me and just listened. I cried harder at first, but I felt less alone. Once I stopped crying, I was able to visit with my friend who stayed for a short while.

There were times when some staff were unsure about what to do when I broke down. After watching helplessly for a few seconds, one therapist ignored my sobbing and made me complete a task. This was an awful experience. When my distress was ignored, I felt even more embarrassed about breaking down in a room full of strangers. It's difficult to know how to comfort someone you don't know well, but Michelle and Bobbie used two different strategies that worked for me.

I was surprised by how many times a day everyone stopped paying attention to this repetitively used phrase. In the first two weeks my PT insisted that I was getting better, but I was depressed because nothing got easier. Being a therapist myself didn't help. I couldn't look down at my body to analyze what I was doing while I was doing it. It turns out that Michelle was helping me less and less so walking was getting harder because I was gradually doing more of the work. I had done the same thing when I was a therapist and didn't explain what I was doing to my clients either.

Saving My Sanity on the Weekends

Five hours of therapy each day kept me busy during the week, but therapy stops on the weekends. Network TV on the weekends is really bad. You don't actually think hospitals have cable TV. My visitors didn't fill up the long hours of free time. As I stared at the ceiling for hours, time went by so slowly that each weekend was an agony to be endured. Recreational therapy saved my sanity.

When Kathy visited my room and said she could help me play solitaire, I jumped at the opportunity to work on my sitting **endurance** and the coordination in my left arm. I enjoyed playing solitaire as a child but hadn't played it for years. Kathy lent me a deck of cards and a deck shuffler so I could play one-handed. At first, I could play for only fifteen minutes because holding my head and trunk upright was so exhausting. My uncoordinated left hand knocked the rows crooked every time I reached for a card. Yet I kept playing because I got caught up in wanting to win, even if I had to cheat.

Kathy helped me do other meaningful activities I was interested in. While reading has been a life-long leisure activity, holding a book or magazine one-handed was tiring because my sound hand never got a break. Kathy lent me a book rest and I was eventually able to read for two hours at a time, which made the weekends fly by. When she discovered that I'd done crossword puzzles all my life, she xeroxed large crossword puzzles so I could practice printing with my non-dominant hand. Writing was important to me because I wanted to write my own checks and manage my own financial affairs again. Doing large crossword puzzles was a fun way to practice writing. It forced me to think and was more interesting than just copying letters. Recreational therapy is a powerful adjunct to the other therapies in a rehabilitation hospital, especially on the weekends.

Dealing with the Hospital System

The way a hospital is run is annoying, but I had the advantage of knowing how the system works. Patients aren't allowed to do even simple things, like use the toilet, without a doctor's written permission. There is no point in arguing with the nurses. They are just following the doctor's orders. When I wanted something, I asked my doctor to write orders that stated what I was allowed to do. My doctor was reluctant to grant my request to shower, so he had me evaluated by an OT. She talked my doctor into giving me showering privileges with supervision. My OT was an advocate in other ways, too. Leslie sent an order to dietary to put a rocker knife on my tray with every meal. This adapted knife allowed me to cut my food one-handed instead of letting it get cold while I waited for someone to cut it up for me.

Having worked as a nurse's aide before I went to college, I knew not to make a request at the end or beginning of a shift. Shifts usually change at 7:00 a.m., 3:00 p.m., and 11:00 p.m. New staff coming on duty aren't free to answer call buttons because they have to attend a meeting to learn how clients did on the last shift. Staff who are going off shift don't want to start a task they can't finish before it's time to go home. Here is an example of how I made the system work for me. I was most successful when I asked for a **shower** at 5:00 a.m. This gave the aide assigned to me time to rearrange her workload so she could go into the shower with me at 6:00 a.m. Then she could stay with me until I finished showering without having to stay past the end of her shift at 7:00 a.m.

Even though I had worked in a rehabilitation hospital, I didn't know that nursing staff feel stressed out by their large caseloads and some aides work double shifts to make ends meet. A simple way to get busy staff to help me was to call them by their names instead of "nurse." I didn't know the names of every nurse and aide, but I made the effort to learn the names of the nice ones. Instead of sending impersonal store-bought thank-you cards, I typed individual letters on the computer in recreational therapy that described specifically how four nursing staff had helped me. I gave the letters to the nursing supervisor who showed the letters to the nurses and put them in their files. At the facility I was in, nursing staff who are singled out for providing good care are given an award and a $200 prize. I think personalized thank-you notes mean more than the flowers and boxes of candy that nurses often receive.

Setting the Stage for Success

My recovery was influenced by two powerful beliefs. I already knew about the power of persistence. It had been a thrill to see what some of the clients I had treated achieved, yet I was stunned by the obstacles that persistence helped me overcome. By persistence I don't mean determination, which is an intention, but a willingness to repeat one's actions. When I try something new, I frequently fail on the first attempt. Sometimes postponing my second attempt is helpful. I don't remember what mistakes I made yesterday, so I discover solutions by doing the task differently the next day. Happy accidents are as much a part of my recovery as my advanced training in stroke rehabilitation. My frustration is less intense the next day, which allows me to see that I get stronger, faster, and more coordinated when I repeat a movement. I eventually learned not to judge how successful I would be from my first attempt. My belief in the power of persistence is based on observable success.

The second factor that profoundly influenced my recovery was a change in my belief about the loving kindness of people. I had thought that the generosity I'd seen portrayed in movies was idealistic. I received help from fourteen people. Where would I be now if my friends and family hadn't come to my rescue? Their help propelled me towards independence so I could go home again. Yet it was hard for me to accept all of this kindness. I still saw myself as a therapist who helped others and a divorcée who had learned how to take care of herself. When an independent person suddenly feels helpless, it is easy to fall into a pattern of complaining or criticizing. I knew my reaction to feeling helpless would create an emotional climate that influenced how people treated me. Knowing that I was doing everything I could do made it easier for me to be gracious about accepting help with things I couldn't do. Being as grateful as you can at the moment is both selfish and kind.

I paid attention to what people **volunteered** for. They offered to help with tasks they enjoy or could do with the least inconvenience. Listening to what they were willing to do worked out better than trying to guess whom I should ask to help with a specific task. Having small groups of people get together to decide how to help me was more successful than shanghaiing one poor soul who would quickly be overwhelmed. Loving kindness is powerful, but asking one person to care for a stroke survivor is setting up that person for failure.

The Bottom Line

The procedures in this book are written in enough detail so people who don't know how to do them can visualize what I'm talking about. Have you ever read instructions on how to put something together only to find that some steps were left out? Skipping steps is a surefire way to confuse readers and make them think it's their fault.

When I mention equipment, I give you websites and store names. You may not have the exact store I mention near you, but it is good to use non-medical sources for ADL equipment. Anything sold in a medical catalogue is usually more expensive. Retail stores have discovered that senior citizens want adapted equipment.

However, procedures and equipment don't take into account that a stroke happens to a person. A new procedure or piece of equipment can trigger anger or grief instead of enthusiasm. Because I learned so long ago what each ADL task requires, I am often startled and upset when I learn that my stroke disrupts yet another ADL. So before describing a solution, I talk about the impact the problem had on my life. Seeing how a problem can affect your life may help you understand why you might want to change lifelong habits and learn how to do tasks a new way.

When people disagree about what ADL tasks a stroke survivor *should* do, remember the meaning of a task is personal. It's not how difficult a new procedure is that determines if you will learn it; it's what the task means to you. If a stroke survivor resents having his or her mail opened, a caregiver may have to learn to watch a loved one struggle without interfering. Stroke survivors may gain independence in a task because it frees the people they love to do activities without being constantly interrupted. Independence is a social contract that has to be renegotiated after you have a stroke. Don't assume you know what the other person wants.

Before you get engrossed in reading about procedures and equipment, remember that people cannot be reprogrammed like robots. After you and your family have talked, locate the topics you want to revisit by using the Table of Contents or the Index. The Index contains key words that are spread out over more than one chapter. Key words are **printed in bold** in the text.

As you read, keep in mind that how one person succeeds doesn't always work for another person. I am particularly concerned about safety issues for stroke survivors who have different deficits than I do because their stroke affected a different part of the brain. A few examples of deficits that can affect safety are the inability to understand multi-step directions, poor safety awareness, poor hot/cold discrimination, and unilateral neglect. Unilateral neglect is a lack of awareness of the hemiplegic side or even all objects on one side of the body. Therefore, I have underlined a few safety issues in the chapters to come when stroke survivors and their caretakers need to be extra vigilant.

It's hard to think clearly during the first month after a stroke when everyone is experiencing shock and grief. It's also hard to express your concerns to the health care team when you don't know what they are yet. It's easier to identify concerns if you have a better understanding of how a stroke affects your ability to stay in your home. I hope this book helps you think ahead and speak up. While therapists have the formal training and experience with other stroke survivors that you lack, you know more about your situation than they do. When baby boomers overwhelm the health care system, stroke survivors and their families who are proactive will have more options.

References

American Heart Association. *Heart Disease and Stroke Statistics–2007 Update*. http://circ.ahajournals.org.

CHAPTER 2

REGAINING MOBILITY

When you say "I want to walk again" you are making a commitment to work on strength, balance, and endurance. Regaining mobility includes learning to wrestle with the bed linen and putting good lighting on the stairs to prevent a fall. Regaining mobility takes persistence because mobility issues appear again and again. Just when I think I've licked a mobility issue, it pops up in a new situation. Fortunately, living in a wheelchair for two months helped me see that all the hard work is worth it.

Regaining mobility means learning to overcome bad habits. Just as a car depreciates the minute you drive it off the lot, the skills you learn in the hospital start fading at the curb. A theme that repeats throughout this chapter is my struggle to undo bad habits after they have caused an injury. **Memory aids**, such as a mental picture or verbal cue, can help you remember to move safely. However, memory aids are personal. What works for me may not work for you. My examples illustrate what a memory aid is good for rather than serving as a rulebook that will work for everyone. The key to success is creating a "do" instead of a "don't." It's a waste of time to remind yourself not to do something because you still have to figure out what you should do instead. Finding memory aids that work for you may take time, but pain is a great teacher.

Bed Mobility is a Burden

Not being able to move around in bed was one of the challenges I resented the most. Bed mobility was a burden because it required energy at night when I was the most tired. It initially took twice as many moves to change my position in bed as it used to. For example, I preferred getting out of bed by rolling onto my sound side because I could use my sound arm to push myself up to sitting. However, I couldn't just roll onto my side. To **prevent a fall**, I had to scoot away from the edge of the bed while on my back so I wouldn't fall off the bed when I rolled over. Then when I rolled onto my sound side, my floppy right arm would get stuck behind me. It literally felt like a wrestler was pinning me to the bed. I had to remember to use my sound hand to pull my hemiplegic arm across my chest *before* I started to roll. It was aggravating to know that I used to roll over in bed with one complex movement.

Another bed mobility issue is scooting up in bed. It's fun to work the controls that make the head of a hospital bed go up and down until you discover that you've slid down in bed and your back is now where your hips are supposed to be. I already knew how to scoot up by bridging, so I thought I had it made. Bridging involves bending your knees while lying on your back, pushing your hips up in the air, and using both feet to shove your body up towards the head of the bed. I quickly learned that, unlike the mat tables clients sit on for therapy, a bed has linen that creates a lot of friction. To help overcome the friction that linens create when I bridge to scoot up in bed, I reach overhead with my sound hand to pull on the top of the mattress. It's hard for a family to take someone home who is dead weight in the bed, so scooting up in bed is a good trick to learn.

My OT evaluated my bed mobility by asking me to lie down on top of a bedspread and sit back up, but I learned that this is really mat table mobility. Bed mobility includes moving bed linens out of the way so you don't end up lying on top of them. When I moved around in bed, I often got the bed linens pinned under my hemiplegic side. Trying to pull the sheet and blanket out from under me was like wrestling a boa constrictor. I tried to get my hemiplegic side off of the bed linens by rolling onto my sound side, but the linens were behind me where I couldn't reach them. The only way I could get off the linens was to get out of bed, move the linens where I wanted them, and get back in bed.

Suddenly, seven months after my stroke, I learned to turn over in bed in either direction and handle the covers without waking up. I don't know what I'm doing differently because I learned it in my sleep. So don't give up on your hopes for a good night's sleep. As a therapist, I had never asked my clients to get under the covers and wrestle with the bed linens so it never dawned on me to ask my OT to help me with this task. Learn from my mistake. Ask your OT to evaluate bed mobility at bedside where moving around under the covers comes into play.

Standing Up and Going Floppo

When I was a therapist, I thought that standing up was easier if your body weight was equally divided between both legs. Boy, was I wrong. Imagine my surprise when I learned that using both legs to stand up is hard for someone with a stroke. It was actually easier to put most of my weight on my sound leg. At first it was easier because my sound leg always responded first. My hemiplegic leg was like a child who ignores a command until you get in the child's face and firmly repeat the instruction over and over. It's discouraging and exhausting to concentrate this hard on a leg that is unable to cooperate at first. While my PT made sure I knew how to stand up by putting some weight on my hemiplegic leg, I didn't do what she taught me when I got home. The bad habit of putting most of my weight on my sound leg returned because my sound leg is so strong it's freaky.

Michelle made sure I sat down slowly by watching me like a predator watches its prey. Sitting down badly didn't become a problem until I went home and had access to upholstered furniture. I quickly developed the bad habit of going "floppo" by leaning back and letting myself fall on to the couch or bed. As a therapist I knew better, but I did it anyway. This bad habit eventually transferred to hard surfaces like the **toilet**, so plopping down was beating up my spine. I tried to break myself of this habit by standing up when I went "floppo" and then sitting down correctly, but that didn't change my behavior the next time I sat down.

I was sorry I let myself develop these bad habits because I re-injured my back. People with sore backs may wonder why people with back spasms don't just suck it up. In addition to the intense pain, panic sets in because almost every motion involves the back. Rolling over in bed can trigger back spasms. The slightest leg movement can be painful because you rely on your stomach and back muscles to help lift your leg. The worst news is that almost every back muscle is attached to the rib cage, so even breathing stresses the back muscles.

Take my word for it, you don't want to have back spasms after you've had a stroke. If I was walking when the spasms began, I had to stand still, lean on my cane, bear the agony, and hope I wouldn't fall down. Bending over to sit down on the toilet was so painful that it was hard to relax enough to go to the bathroom. When I finished PT for my back, I became a fanatic about sitting down and standing up slowly with my feet parallel. When your hemiplegic foot doesn't point straight ahead, you automatically put more weight on your sound leg. This asymmetrical **position** twists the spine and overuses certain back muscles, which can become tight.

Here are **memory aids** that helped me stop going "floppo" and standing up incorrectly. To sit down, I keep my hemiplegic arm close to my hemiplegic leg as I reach for my shoe. My hemiplegic hand doesn't actually touch my leg or shoe, but this visual cue reminds me to (1) look down to see if both feet are pointed forwards, (2) lean forwards instead of backwards, and (3) put weight on both feet as I bend both knees. To stand up, I place my fisted hemiplegic hand on my thigh and straighten my elbow. My hemiplegic arm doesn't provide much assistance, but the pressure on my thigh is a tactile cue that reminds me to put weight on my hemiplegic leg.

You may not have a bad back like I do. You may have arthritis in your neck, bad knees, or an old sports injury. People often have joints that are stiff or achy before they have a stroke. Going "floppo" and standing up with contortions can re-injure a part of your body that is already vulnerable. Therapists are the safety police because they don't want you to fall on their watch. You have to take over this role when you go home. Have you developed harmful ways of standing up or sitting down since coming home that put you at risk? What memory aids do you need to use to protect your body when you stand up and sit down? Agony is a magnificent teacher, but I can't recommend it.

If you are short, standing up is especially difficult after you've had a stroke. I feel like a badger living in a land of long-legged gazelles. If Americans sat on the floor, I'd have it made. Regrettably, adult furniture is too deep from front to back to accommodate a five-foot two-inch person. I don't want to perpetually perch on the edge of furniture so I slide back in the seat so I have some back support. When

I slide back like this, my *toes* touch the floor but my *heels* hover about an inch above the floor. To stand up, I have to scoot to the edge of the furniture until my knees are over my toes. I challenge tall people to sit on the edge of a bed, scoot back until the back of your calves are touching the bed, and then try to stand up.

Scooting forward got me in trouble. My therapists thought I didn't have good safety awareness, which was embarrassing. It took me a few days to figure out what I was doing that made them so nervous. Since I've had to scoot forward before standing up all my life I didn't think about the signal this was giving my therapists. I knew I was going to stop at the edge of the furniture and wait for my therapists to tell me when to stand up, but they didn't know that. I fixed this problem by watching my therapists' faces and not moving a muscle until they were ready. I had to reassure them in this way for a couple of weeks to regain their confidence. If your tall therapist doesn't like the way you stand up, it might help to explain how being "height challenged" adds to your dilemma.

Wheelchairs Can Wreck a Home

Once I could transfer to the wheelchair, I was hell on wheels. I eventually pushed myself all around the rehab hospital. I made the mistake of mentioning how hard it was to propel the wheelchair by digging with my sound heel and pushing the wheel rim with my sound hand. My therapist got me a super-low wheelchair so I was closer to the ground. I could stand up with less effort and got better traction when I propelled the wheelchair with my heel. I was thrilled with the super-low wheelchair until I found out that I could barely get my chin over the top of the bathroom sink while brushing my teeth in sitting. Be careful what you wish for.

It was relatively easy to keep the **wheelchair** going straight down a wide hospital hallway, but I learned to maneuver around furniture in my room by banging into everything. Even in a large hospital room, my roommates and I bumped into the same furniture over and over again. I crashed into furniture because wheelchair parts stick out in every direction. It's easier to maneuver a wheelchair when there are no leg rests to catch on the furniture. A legless chair also has a smaller turning radius. I learned to take the leg rests off as soon as I got back to my room. At first, I had to hold my hemiplegic leg up by crossing my sound leg under it when I propelled the chair across the room. I eventually learned to propel my wheelchair around my hospital room by alternately digging with my sound and hemiplegic heel.

An extra long brake handle on the hemiplegic side is a blessing and a curse. The sound hand doesn't have to reach as far across the body to lock the brake. However, this long brake handle sticks out so far that it catches on everything. I knocked a whole row of cards off as I wheeled past a card rack in a store on an outing with recreational therapy. When I got back to the hospital, I asked for a regular brake handle on my hemiplegic side. It was worth the extra effort to reach farther across my body to push the shorter brake handle with my sound hand.

It's especially difficult to propel a wheelchair backwards though doorways. When my roommates and I backed out of the bathroom, we would hit the doorjamb several times before we lined up the wheelchair just right. Looking back over your shoulder isn't very effective. You are clear on one side, but not on the other. A roommate taught me that it was easier to turn the wheelchair around inside the large hospital bathroom and come out forwards. I never backed out of the hospital bathroom after I learned this maneuver. If you have bathrooms at home that are too small to turn a wheelchair around in, you are going to be very frustrated until you learn to back the wheelchair out so slowly that it is like watching honey slide down the side of a jar.

Clients who have to go home with a wheelchair will gouge their own furniture and doorways. All you have to do is look at the gouges on the doors and walls of every room in a rehab hospital to see that maneuvering a wheelchair with one arm and one leg is difficult. If you know you are going home with a wheelchair, practice moving the wheelchair slowly around every obstacle while you are in the hospital.

Squats are Your Friend

My PT had me squat down in standing to pick up cones on a footstool with my sound hand and stand up to place the cones on a ledge that was as high as I could reach. Michelle had me do this almost every day and I never got tired of it. If she didn't do it in the morning, I asked her to do it in the afternoon. I loved stacking cones because I felt safe while I succeeded at a task that challenged my standing balance – a deficit that frightened me badly. I acquired excellent balance while squatting, but I had to use my OT training to apply this motor skill to ADLs.

To be more accurate, ADLs require mini-squats where you bend your knees only a few inches. The first benefit of mini-squats I discovered was to bend down to pull up my pants while standing at the **toilet**. **Handling underwear** with one hand is frustrating because underwear sticks to sweaty skin. It's also awkward to reach behind you to pull the waistband up over your hemiplegic hip. My **balance** was better when I reached down to grab my pants by bending both knees and hips instead of leaning forward by jackknifing at the hips. When I shared this discovery with my PT, she was glad she wasn't an OT who has to do toilet training.

Unfortunately, nurses' aides do toilet training. They solve mobility problems by providing maximum physical assistance whether or not it is needed. I was shocked the first time an aide pulled my underpants up and down without being asked. Nurses' aides have big caseloads so they are trying to get to the next client as quickly as possible. I wonder how many families get a nasty surprise when they are told a family member is independent in self-care only to find out they have to wait on their loved one hand-and-foot in the bathroom. It's not our fault. It took me weeks of asking the nursing staff every day on every shift to let me pull my pants up and down. They finally relented and called me "Miss Independent."

In addition to helping with toileting, mini-squats are helpful during morning care at the sink if you are confined to a wheelchair. When I bathed at the sink, the only way to wash my crotch without soaking my foam seat cushion was to stand up. For safety, I locked the brakes and kept the wheelchair close behind me so I had a place to sit down quickly. To get a washcloth and towel between my legs to wash and dry my crotch, I spread my feet a few inches apart and did a mini-squat. I also felt safer if I did a mini-squat as I stood to lean over to wash my face with my eyes closed and spit out toothpaste.

Mini-squats make it easier to **handle clothing** when I shower at home. I walk into my bathroom wearing a T-shirt and underpants. Even though I have a chair next to the tub, I don't want to pull down my underpants, sit down, and put one of the dirtiest parts of my body on a chair to pull my feet out of the leg holes. I stand and lower my underpants until they drop to the ground. <u>For safety, I hold on</u> to the sink as I step out of my underpants and do a mini-squat to pick them up off the floor. <u>For safety, you may need to use</u> a reacher or have someone pick up your underpants. However you do it, dropping your underpants to the floor is safer than trying to take step out of them while you are standing. Stroke survivors are taught to dress while sitting on the edge of the bed, but we also need to learn how to **prevent falls** while handle clothing in the bathroom.

Mini-squats even turned out to be handy during **cane retrieval**. Stroke survivors have to retrieve their canes dozens of times after they go home. Quad canes have four prongs so they stay put on linoleum, but they often fall over on carpeting. Leaning a single-point cane against a piece of furniture is risky. It can fall down even after it has stayed in place for several minutes. I was unaware of this daily aggravation when I was in the hospital because my cane was handed to me when I walked and taken away from me when I finished. Waiting for a caregiver to pick up your cane and hand it to you gets old for both parties. While a long-handled reacher can be clipped to a cane, it doesn't do you any good when it is attached to a cane that has fallen out of your reach. I would make a fortune if I could get paid to pick up other people's canes.

If doing mini-squats to retrieve a cane <u>is not safe for you</u>, here are three alternatives. First, beat gravity to the punch by putting your cane on the floor near your feet where you can reach it. An example is putting your cane under your seat at a concert. Second, wedge your cane between two pieces of furniture. An example is wedging your cane between a table and a chair. Third, lean a cane against a wall where people won't trip over it. For example, ask a companion to lean your cane against the wall when you go to a restaurant. The waitress may not see you cane when she gets close to serve you. I don't know if training stroke survivors to safely retrieve a fallen cane is OT's or PT's job, but cane management should be a regular part of rehab training.

Balance Skills You Need at Home

Laying the groundwork in the hospital. As good as my balance was during squats where both feet were on the ground, it was terrible when I had to walk. My PT was good at catching me and pulling me upright, but I was hysterical because I couldn't feel myself falling. I was freaked out because I couldn't fix mistakes I couldn't feel. All I could think about at this early stage of gait training was that I'd end up in a wheelchair. Yet there was no way I could go home in a wheelchair to a two-story house with one bathroom on the second floor.

After a few weeks of gait training, I noticed that the toes of my hemiplegic foot curled up when I leaned too far in one direction. I learned to pay attention to how much weight was on the borders of each foot as I stepped onto it. Too much weight on my toes or heels meant I was leaning too far forward or backward. Too much weight on one side of my foot or the other meant I was leaning too far to one side. I also learned to look straight ahead. It's easier to stay upright when I look at a vertical image, like a wall. Even furniture will do. I finally had early warning signs that I was starting to fall. The power of persistence, learning to compensate with visual input and sensory feedback from my feet, and the help of a talented PT produced a miracle. After eight weeks, I could walk independently with a quad cane. I thought the majority of my balance problems were over.

Going home. I quickly learned that going home presents a whole new set of balance challenges. This insight was forcefully brought home on the first day when I fell down a full flight of stairs. I could see the wall passing by me as I fell backwards from the top of stairs, but I had absolutely no sensation of falling. I fell backwards, landed on my back, and somersaulted heels-over-head to the bottom of the stairs. I was completely limp, which is probably why I didn't break any bones. That night as I was falling asleep, I felt the sensation of falling for about two seconds, but it stopped abruptly and I've never had nightmares about that fall. If you told me a story like this, I wouldn't believe you, but it happened to me so I know it is true. After this bad fall, I wouldn't have had the courage to face my balance problems without the encouragement and expertise of my home health PT.

The first balance challenge that Lincoln addressed was climbing stairs. In the PT gym, a continuous railing wraps around all sides at the top of the practice stairs. When I stood at the top of the stairs at home, the railing was behind me where I couldn't reach it any more. When this happens, Lincoln taught me that doorjambs are my friend. To **prevent a fall**, he taught me to reach over and grab the bathroom doorjamb at the top of the stairs *before* I stepped up onto the top step. I also learned to grab the doorjamb of the front door of the house before I step outside. Unlike railings, doorjambs are everywhere. Keep your eyes peeled because you will feel safer whenever you see a doorjamb.

A second balance challenge at home was maneuvering in tight spaces. Here are two examples. First, after closing the bathroom door and **flushing the toilet** I had to turn around by pivoting 180 degrees in place. Second, maneuvering through the narrow space between my friend's couch and coffee table without getting my **cane** caught required concentration. Arlene offered to get rid of the coffee table, but my PT decided that the table was far enough from the couch for my ability level. Leaving the coffee table where it was gave me experience I needed. I didn't want to ask people to "Rebecca-proof" their homes every time I came to visit. I didn't want to be homebound because I couldn't maneuver in other people's homes. Walking in straight lines in a big open therapy gym doesn't prepare you to maneuver in tight spaces at home. Ask your home health PT to teach you to turn 180 degrees in the bathroom. Look around your home to see if furniture needs to be moved to help you **prevent a fall** in tight spaces.

A third balance challenge was learning to stop suddenly. A large PT gym has plenty of room to maneuver in so you don't have to stop suddenly to avoid obstacles. When an occasional traffic jam forms, therapists stop their clients and make sure the slowest client passes first. Expect situations at home that require you to stop quickly, like children or pets who aren't watching where they are going. I had to contend with two cats who were afraid of my **cane**. I learned to stop quickly whenever I saw the cats and wait until they steeled their nerves to dash around me. Identify when you have to stop suddenly at home. Ask your home health PT to help you practice stopping quickly to **prevent a fall**.

I fell several times in the first month before I mastered these basic balance skills. All my falls were before breakfast or at bedtime, yet I could walk safely for several days during these times. Then I would fall without warning, like a driver who is driving on dry pavement and suddenly finds himself hydroplaning. To my surprise, my perceived level of exhaustion is not a good predictor I can use to **prevent a fall**. I can feel exhausted but walk safely one night and feel pleasantly tired the next night but start stumbling as soon as I get up to go to bed.

I fell one night after walking to the bathroom safely for a month. My home health PT suggested a bedside commode. I refused to buy one because I had to be ready to live alone. I didn't see how I was going to **transport**, empty, and clean a commode. Then serendipity gave me the opportunity to choose more wisely. If only I had known then what I know now about walking aids.

Canes, Walkers, Braces, and Shoes

A second stroke taught me when to use **different types of walking aids**. This time I had to go home with a hemi-walker, which is a walker with a handle in the center of the crossbar so you can lift it with your sound hand. After two weeks at home, I no longer needed the hemi-walker during the day, but I still used it to **walk to the bathroom** at night and take a shower in the morning. Using a walker to go to the bathroom was definitely better than using a bedside commode. The walker slowed me down, but I didn't mind because I was half asleep. Even though I've recovered enough to use a single-point cane during the day, I use my quad cane to go to the bathroom at night and shower in the morning.

I continued to use this tiered use of walking aids when I was ready to walk in the community. I initially used a quad cane when I walked in a store that required maneuvering around obstacles. The four prongs gave me more stability and made people stay farther away from me. I initially used a single-point cane outdoors only when I walked in low-traffic areas, like walking around my block.

Having a variety of walking aids to meet the demands of different times of day and different settings lets you use the one that gives you the support you need. Save every piece of walking equipment you buy. Talk to your home health PT about which device is best for each setting that you want to be mobile in.

Also save every leg brace. After two years of walking in the community, my current leg brace broke while I was in a restaurant. With a few stumbles, I was able to get home safely where I immediately put on the brace that had been made a week after my first stroke. This old brace didn't fit well because my calf and foot were swollen when it was made. It is common for the lower extremity to swell when people stop walking because walking massages body fluids out of the legs. I had to walk more slowly with this looser brace, but I was able to walk safely for the week that it took Wayne, my brace man, to fix the other brace. If you need to wear a leg brace, get to know your brace man. He will keep you walking long after therapy ends.

Walking aids also include shoes. After a year of walking safely in the house while wearing my leg brace but not using a cane, I had two bad falls. I fell hard and was on the floor faster than I thought possible. The fear of ending up in a wheelchair came back to haunt me, so I asked my doctor to send me to a PT who was trained in myofascial release. This treatment approach teaches therapists to evaluate and treat poor body alignment. After putting her thumbs on my two hip bones, Tracy decided I had acquired a leg-length discrepancy from a shoe salesman. Because the thickness of a leg brace adds length to the hemiplegic leg, this shoe salesman had developed the habit of putting two sole inserts inside the shoe that goes on the sound foot. However, **shoe inserts** in orthopedic shoes have a raised edge, which adds a lot of height when doubled. With one leg longer than the other, I had developed a lurch that kept throwing me off **balance**.

Tracy decided that the only insert I needed under my sound leg to make my two legs equal in length was one thin Dr. Scholl's pad. My balance was better as soon as I stood up with this thinner insert. Tracy was the only person who talked to me about shoe inserts. My shoes get constant wear because of the limited shoe selection that fits over my brace. Before you leave the hospital, learn about the correct shoe inserts so you know what to do the next time you buy a new pair of shoes.

Multitasking Means Having a Life

As my balance improved, I gained the ability to multitask while walking. **Multitasking** is the ability to divide your attention. During walking, it refers to how much you can trust your hemiplegic leg to do what it's supposed to do while you focus on something else. The ability to multitask gives you access to your heart and mind while you control your body. Stroke survivors have to talk while we are standing. We have to make decisions while we are reaching. Yet I was taught to walk, talk, and manipulate objects in three separate rooms by three different therapists. This division of labor creates gaps in mobility training that I wasn't aware of until I went home.

At first, I couldn't divide my attention at all. For example, I made the mistake of thinking about what I wanted to wear as I was taking a step. Boom! I went down like a tree. For weeks I had been taking that step toward the clothesbasket at the head of the bed where I temporarily kept my clothes at my friend's house. I thought it was safe to think about what I wanted to wear instead of concentrating on what my hemiplegic leg was doing. In that instant, I forgot to make sure that my hemiplegic foot was flat before I put weight on it.

My home health PT thought I was high functioning because I could walk independently with a cane and leg brace. Yet walking by devoting all my attention to my hemiplegic leg was depressing. For me, walking means being able to do activities that are useful or fun. Walking got easier, but it was hard for me to keep a positive attitude about my success. I wanted to be more than a body that moved around the house with a brain that couldn't afford to think about anything but a leg.

When my home health PT started to have me walk outside, it was impossible to multitask at first. Walking down the main street of a small town was as disorienting as walking through a haunted house at an amusement park. I had to constantly look down at the sidewalk that was sloped to make the rain run off and watch for sections of concrete that were heaved up. Initially I had to stop every time I looked in a store window, every time I looked for cars before crossing a street, and every time someone spoke to me. What a nightmare! Walking outside is much harder than walking around the inpatient gym where you've memorized the location of every piece of equipment and the floor is flat and level. My home health PT kept walking me outside day after day until I got better. I knew my ability to multitask had improved when I looked up without stumbling as a friend drove by and yelled hello.

It is still difficult for me to have more than a predictable chat while I'm standing or walking (e.g., "How are you?" "I'm fine, and you?"). During a more complex conversation, it takes too much of my attention to process what the other person is saying and figure out how to respond if I am standing. It turns out that compensating for **poor balance** is costly. While listening to the other person, I have to feel if my weight is evenly distributed on both feet and glance at vertical images to see if I'm leaning away from vertical. It's not that I'm thinking about my balance every second. It's more like waiting for the results of a medical test. You're not consciously thinking about the test, but when the results come back you suddenly realize how much you've been worrying. I'm not aware of how much mental energy I am using to monitor my balance until I sit down and breathe a sigh of relief.

I was horrified when I finally understood why I kept asking friends for advice or help when we were sitting around a table to eat. I could see that people didn't appreciate it when I inserted my issues into a meal situation. It took me two years to figure out why I kept doing this. I realize now that I refused to tell people about my balance problem because I could not accept that it would never be normal again. I had developed superb balance as a child while learning to pirouette on my toes in ballet. As an adult, I enjoyed activities that required the ability to make sudden turns, like downhill skiing, skating, and Scottish country dancing. In the end, it was painful to let poor balance interfere with social grace. I am finally able to tell people I need to sit down to talk about something and let the person choose when he or she wants to talk. If you have trouble talking, using your hemiplegic hand, or making a decision while you are standing or walking, consider sitting down.

The Most Dangerous Room is the Kitchen

Many people think the bathroom is the most dangerous room in the house, but bathrooms have safety equipment, like grab bars. Once you transfer to the shower chair, you are going to be there for a while. For me, the kitchen is the most dangerous room because it requires advanced balance skills while **multitasking**. After two months I got tired of eating frozen dinners and decided to learn how to cook one-handed while wearing my leg brace. When I tackled a new task for the first time, I often stumbled because I forgot to tell my hemiplegic leg to lift high enough to clear my toes. This initially made me unsafe. I wasn't used to thinking about where my feet were. I was used to thinking about following a recipe and many other aspects of cooking.

Food preparation requires advanced **balance** because you have to repeatedly turn to walk back and forth between the stove, sink, refrigerator, and cupboards. Even a simple task like preparing a sliced banana on cereal and opening a soda requires a lot of turning. I store breakfast supplies close together and do this simple task six days a week, but I've never reduced the number of times I have to turn to less than fifteen. I'm not exaggerating when I say that maneuvering in the kitchen requires dozens of turns in a short period of time.

You don't have to make linguine alfredo to be challenged in the kitchen. Something as ordinary as putting away groceries requires multitasking and good balance. Groceries don't come out of the bag in the order I need them. Using a **rolling cart** makes it easy to quickly get cold food in the refrigerator, but I have to get canned and packaged goods out of my way. I repeatedly turn and take a step to place these items on the counter. Once I roll the cart to the refrigerator, I have to make decisions as I reach down and overhead. Frozen food goes in the freezer, vegetables go in the low bins, and some food at the front of a shelf has to be pushed back to make room. After using the rolling cart to transport canned foods to the proper cabinet, I have to decide where I want them to go and shift my weight to put them there. For example, I lean down to put large cans on the top shelf of a base cabinet that rests on the floor. Small cans go on a turntable in an overhead cabinet. This means reaching to move cans around on the turntable to make room for the new cans. I'm not a fanatic, but I at least like the cans of soup grouped together rather than mixed in with the canned vegetables.

Even the simplest task in the kitchen demands repeated turning, bending, and reaching while making decisions and inspecting your environment. This is what makes the kitchen so dangerous. Ask an OT to teach you how to deal with these challenges. The long, straight walks I took with every one of my PTs didn't prepare me for the kitchen.

Inexpensive Home Modifications Prevent Falls

Home modification can help you **prevent falls**. Don't assume that every home modification is expensive. A relatively simple home modification is to remove hazards that trip people and can cause a fall, like electrical wires and throw rugs.

My second home health OT helped me get rid of clutter that put me at risk for falling. Two years after my first stroke, I could walk through tight spaces with ease because I could walk indoors without a cane. When I went home after my second stroke with a **walker**, I discovered that accumulated clutter tripped me or forced me to lean precariously when I reached for things. My walker got caught in a narrow space that a stack of magazines had created in my home office. Kim moved the magazines from the floor to a table. She moved clutter on the floor of a closet that forced me to move objects every time I reached for objects I use regularly, like a coat. She put a flower stand in my shed because it partially blocked a doorway that made it difficult to get my hemi-walker and the cart loaded with dirty clothes into the laundry room. She helped me distribute the flowers to new locations in the living room. She moved objects off the floor of my shed so I wouldn't have to lean over to reach for items on the shelves. I had made the mistake of asking people to put things in my shed without going with them to keep them from just dropping items inside the door. An OT can quickly improve your safety at home by showing you how to get rid of clutter that creates unnecessary hazards.

For me, walking too fast contributed to two bad falls I had in the kitchen. The speed that works outdoors where I can walk in a straight line crept into the turns I have to make in the kitchen. To **prevent more falls**, I first tried verbal **memory aids**. Repeatedly asking myself if I was turning slowly didn't work. This self-questioning strategy was hard to sustain when food preparation and clean-up lasts for hours each day. Then I tried placing brightly colored construction paper in places where I turn frequently, like on the refrigerator door. That didn't help either. I quickly learned to ignore them like I ignore the pictures on my walls. I finally discovered that making my big kitchen smaller slows me down. When I cook, I create a temporary corridor in my spacious kitchen by placing my **rolling cart** parallel to the kitchen counter. The cart isn't close enough for me to run into, but it creates a corridor that is narrow enough to make me slow down to maneuver carefully. This is a very inexpensive home modification.

Attending a candlelit women's circle taught me that poor lighting can make poor **balance** worse. As I stood up to light my candle, I almost had a bad fall. The archway across from me could have told me where vertical was, but it was in shadow in the candlelit room. I didn't know that my trunk was leaning far to the left until I felt a strong stretch in the muscles on the right side of my trunk and then felt a lot of weight on the outer border of my left foot. I was able to take a quick hop to bring my sound foot back under my body, but I was unnerved by almost falling in front of a group of seated women.

My nighttime routine illustrates how good lighting can **prevent falls**. When I turn the lights off as I walk to my bedroom, walking towards lighted rooms makes a big difference. It means going into the bedroom to turn on a light *before* I start turning off lights in the living room. Back in the living room, I turn to face the lighted room ahead of me and look up before I turn off the light. If I face away from the lighted area as I turn off a light and turn around in the dark, I may stumble. Having a visual image of where vertical is and not turning in the dark made me safer. When you turn off lights, do you think about safety?

I had an electrician install a porch light with a motion detector. When I approach the house at night, the light automatically turns on. I can see the stairs and handrail before I take a step and quickly find the lock and doorknob so I don't fumble when I open the door. Parts and labor cost me $100, but it was money well spent. I have a one-story house so I don't have inside stairs, but good lighting is an easy way to **prevent falls** on indoor stairwells as well. Do you have to navigate up and down dark stairs?

Installing good lighting, removing throw rugs and extension cords that are in your path, and having someone relocate clutter are inexpensive ways to prevent falls. Have you used these strategies to make you safe at home? When you are in a new environment for the first time, do you evaluate the lighting as soon as you step into that space?

Low Endurance is a Deal Breaker

When I run out of energy, whatever promise I've made has to be broken. Paralysis is predictable, but fatigue can show up unexpectedly for a stroke survivor. Normally when muscles fatigue, they hand off the work to other muscles. Paralysis means fewer muscles are available to share the workload. Before my stroke I used to push myself when I was tired. If I do this now, I learn I am exhausted when I lie down and can't get up for an hour or two. Learning how to prevent fatigue has resurfaced again and again.

My first **endurance** challenge came in the hospital. At first, I couldn't hold my head up for more than two hours at a time. I'd come back to my room after two hours of therapy, get into bed, and fall into a dead sleep. It took five weeks before I could sit up in the wheelchair for four hours. I thought I had it made when I could sit up for most of the day and push my wheelchair all over the hospital.

I had to deal with endurance a second time when I left my wheelchair at the hospital curb. Even though I had walked in the PT gym several times a day by the end, I didn't have the endurance to walk around my friend's tiny apartment. Her downstairs consisted of a small living room, a small kitchen, and a powder room. The upstairs had two bedrooms and a bathroom. Yet walking around this small space was exhausting. I came downstairs in the morning and went up at night. My confidence got a boost when I could walk around this small apartment all day without stopping to lie down on the couch.

My endurance was tested a third time when I moved into my new one-story home to live alone. I was frustrated because gains in endurance came so slowly. I could vacuum only one room a day at first. It took five months before I had the endurance to vacuum all three carpeted rooms in my house in a single day. That day was a landmark for me. I finally believed that I could be an independent homemaker again. Yet even now, when I do moderately heavy housework like vacuuming or bringing groceries in from the car, I still have to take a short rest break after each heavy task.

Some people rest by taking naps, but I've always had trouble falling asleep in the middle of the day unless I'm sick. I tried to rest by watching TV, but it turns me into a zombie who can't stop clicking the remote control because there is nothing good on at the moment. Sometimes I rest by reading a book or doing a crossword puzzle but often end up taking a break that lasts for an hour or more without intending to. The best way for me to take a short break is to listen to music. I can stop the CD after ten or twenty minutes and come back to it whenever I want. Instead of staring at the clock and resenting the interruption, I enjoy the music.

Using a timer to take breaks can be aggravating because it usually beeps in the middle of an activity you want to finish. The only time I use a timer is when I'm working on the computer. I can sit at the computer for six hours and even skip meals. Because I can't be trusted to get up and walk around periodically, I set a timer for one hour and place it in the kitchen so I have to get up to turn it off. After turning the timer off, I take a sip of water from a glass I've placed next to the timer. When I find myself resenting this arbitrary interruption, I remind myself that moving around is aerating my brain. Sitting at the computer for extended periods lets blood pool in my legs where it isn't doing me any good. Drinking water is good because my eyes get dry from not blinking as I stare at the computer screen for hours. What methods have you tried to get yourself to take short breaks?

Preventing fatigue means staying active as well as resting. I found my pedometer and use it to keep track of how far I walk from morning to bedtime. The great thing about a pedometer is that I don't have to take long walks outside. Getting up to retrieve an object makes the number of steps I take that day increase. Walking to the bathroom adds to my daily total. I get credit for walking outside to sit on my patio. Being homebound can turn anyone into an invalid because the effects of inactivity creep up on you. How much do you huff and puff after you walk from the car to the front door of a doctor's office or even after you walk across the room? Wearing a pedometer every day at home can reverse that downward trend.

It is easier to put a pedometer on the waistband of your pants or skirt if you use a clothespin. A wooden clothespin slides in and out of the pedometer more easily than a plastic one. Remove the metal coil that holds the clothespin together. Push half of a wooden clothespin into the clip of the pedometer. With the pedometer held open by the clothespin, push the pedometer down on your waistband and pull the clothespin out. Then slide the pedometer along your waistband to one hip where it keeps track of how many times your hip goes up and down.

I maintain my commitment to **endurance** training by focusing on what I gain. Setting my heart on a particular activity keeps me motivated. For example, staying active and taking rest breaks lets me watch evening TV shows instead of going to bed at six o'clock at night. A perk for you might be having the energy to visit with your grandchildren. It might be having the energy to go out to eat with your family after church. Every commitment you make involves endurance. If I let fatigue rob me of the ability to do activities I love, I might as well give up and go to a nursing home. Has fatigue forced you to say "no" to activities that mean a lot to you?

The Bottom Line

When you say "I want to walk again," you have said a mouthful. Feel-good movies about physical disabilities don't show how much work it takes to regain mobility after you go home. As this chapter shows, the number of feet you can walk doesn't address many mobility issues.

To help us regain mobility, home health services need a sea change. It would be ideal if therapists split their total number of visits and different disciplines alternated seeing you instead of overwhelming you when you get home. It would be good to see OT early if you have issues with self-care but reserve some visits to deal with homecare at a later date when you have better **endurance**. It would be good to see PT early to help you get around your house safely but reserve some visits to deal with mobility in the community. Meeting your PT at the mall later in your recovery would boost your confidence about walking around other people and unfamiliar obstacles.

The day will come when it is too much for me to get around my one-story house and my community. However, every month that I stay in my home leaves more money in my retirement fund. The more money I have left at the end of my life, the more options I have about where I get to live. In the meantime, I work hard to stay mobile so I get to do things I love. From where I stand, learning how to get around after a stroke is a win-win situation. Regaining mobility pays off now and it pays off later.

CHAPTER 3

RECOVERY OF AN ARM AND A HAND

You don't have to have a stroke to know what it is like to lose the use of a hand. When you've forgotten to buy the marshmallows that go on top of the yams at Thanksgiving or you don't have the one wrench you need to complete a project, you've experienced task disruption. It doesn't matter how much food is in your cupboard or how many tools are in your toolbox if the one you need is missing. Try to remember the acute sense of frustration you felt as you yelled "oh, no!" This is how stroke survivors who are one-handed feel every day. It doesn't matter that a task is primarily a one-handed task except for the thirty seconds when you need both hands to complete the task. Stroke survivors have many tasks disrupted when someone isn't standing by to help them.

But I'm jumping the gun. It is typical to regain some control of the shoulder and elbow first. If a therapist had told me that an arm can make you more independent even when you can't move your hand, I wouldn't have believed it. It happened to me and I can hardly believe it. So let's start at the beginning.

The Functional Value of the Hemiplegic Arm

I can carry what in my armpit? Okay, so carrying objects in your armpit sounds goofy. When I was a therapist, I would have felt peculiar reporting in a meeting that a client can carry objects in his or her armpit. You can attach a basket to a **walker**, but how do you **transport** an object when your one good hand is tied up handling a cane? Having to repeatedly ask people to retrieve objects for you is like being a dog who has to beg someone to open the door every time it wants to go out. Sometimes a spouse just wants to watch a football game without being interrupted and a stroke survivor just wants to pick up and carry an object without having to wait.

At first, no matter how hard I concentrated, I couldn't stop my hemiplegic arm from letting go of an object I had tucked in my armpit. It was too much to keep track of the muscle tension in my arm while I concentrated on my leg during walking. My first short-term goal was to carry an object in my hemiplegic armpit a few feet. I started by carrying a small throw pillow tucked in my hemiplegic armpit. The fabric provided friction and the pillow landed safely when it fell. The next object I carried was a videotape. My hemiplegic armpit eventually allowed me to carry a cordless phone, mail, dirty clothes to the clothesbasket, a bottle of shampoo from a grocery bag to the shower, and the list goes on.

Being able to carry a book in my armpit is especially meaningful because I love to read. It's painful to stand at the bookcase and stare at a book I want, knowing I have to go look for a small bag to carry it in. While bags can be tied to a walker, they don't stay attached to a cane. When I want a book, it's great to be able to tuck it in my armpit, go to the couch, sit down, and start reading. Think about objects you want to transport. If you can't carry an object in your hemiplegic hand, consider the lowly armpit.

Arm movements can do what? What an arm can do is amazing. To my surprise, small shoulder movements are functional if you keep your elbow fairly straight. The trick is to do tasks in standing so you don't have to lift your arm very high. I was stunned by what I could do by moving my arm in front or in back of my trunk.

Moving your hemiplegic arm slightly *in front of* your trunk while standing is functional. For example, putting an object in a bag is a nightmare. When I put my sound hand in the bag to open it, it closes as soon as I take my hand out the bag. Lifting my arm slightly in front of my trunk allows me to place my entire hemiplegic hand in a bag to hold it open so I can start filling it. This is useful when filling zip-lock storage bags and produce bags at the grocery store. Getting my arm slightly in front of my trunk also enables me to move large, light objects. For example, I can keep a sheet from hitting the floor when I transfer it from the washer to the dryer by reaching forward and catching the sheet on my hemiplegic forearm.

Moving your hemiplegic arm slightly *behind* your trunk while standing is functional. When my friend took a shower before I did, the wet shower liner would cling to me as I got out of the shower. I used my hemiplegic shoulder and elbow to push the shower liner back as I held on to the grab bar with my sound hand. I could eventually hold the heavy screen door open at my friend's house. I let the screen door close gently on my leg brace while I stepped into the house with my sound leg. I released the door pressing on my brace by reaching back with my hemiplegic arm and pushing the door backwards one inch. The wheelchair-width door at my new home is too heavy for me to use this strategy, but I'm still glad I learned to reach back behind me. I hope these examples of how small arm movements can make you independent give you an idea of what your hemiplegic shoulder and elbow can do.

Why do they make you lean on your hemiplegic arm? Infants strengthen their arms by pushing up on both elbows while lying on their stomachs. When my OT put me on my stomach, I was pleasantly surprised to find that I could push up on both elbows. I was less pleased when I sat up and felt my low backache because this position had forced me to arch my back. Even though I've had years of ballet training, age has finally taken a toll on my flexibility.

So my OT switched tactics. Leslie had me sit on the edge of a mat table and lean to one side to put weight on my hemiplegic elbow. Leaning so far to one side to get my elbow down to the surface of the mat table put a lot of strain on my trunk. Putting a pillow under my elbow so I wouldn't have to bend over as far made me feel insecure. It felt like I was leaning on a wobbly, half-inflated ball.

When my OT asked me to push myself up to sitting by straightening my hemiplegic arm, I failed. I never regained enough strength in the muscle that straightens the hemiplegic elbow to do this. You may want to regain this skill if you prefer sleeping on the side of the bed that forces you to roll onto your hemiplegic side to get up.

I found two instances where leaning on my elbow in standing is useful. I feel safer when I lean down to wash my face with my eyes closed if I steady myself by placing my hemiplegic elbow on the bathroom sink. Leaning on my elbow is also helpful when I take out the trash. The only way I can unlock the lid on my garbage can is to lean my hemiplegic elbow on the lid to hold it still as my sound hand pulls on the handle to lock and unlock it.

I am ambivalent about asking adults to lean on their hemiplegic elbow. While leaning on your elbow strengthens a lot of muscles, there is a limited repertoire of functional activities adults can do in this position. As anyone who has played similar sports like tennis and ping-pong knows, motor control is task specific. Will leaning on your elbow transfer to a useful task? Talk to your OT about this aspect of your treatment. I had to use my OT knowledge to make leaning on my elbow worthwhile.

My PT took a different approach by having me lean on an extended arm. Michelle had me sit on the edge of the mat table with an armchair in front of me. She used an Ace bandage to wrap my hemiplegic hand to one armrest and had me place my sound hand on the other armrest. She helped me stand up and when I felt weight come onto my arms, the muscles that straighten my elbows kicked in. Next she had me shift my weight from side to side while leaning on both armrests so my elbows had to alternately bend and straighten. Leaning on my elbow in *sitting* didn't stimulate the muscle that straightens the elbow (triceps) the way that leaning on both extended arms in *standing* did. This is important because the muscle that bends the elbow (biceps) usually develops too much strength and overpowers the triceps after a stroke.

Unlike leaning on the elbow, leaning on an extended arm while standing has many uses. Even able-bodied adults extend their arm and put a hand out to steady themselves during difficult tasks. An example would be holding on to a ladder while painting the exterior of a house. I initially needed help to maintain my **balance** during simple tasks. Just brushing my teeth could make me wobble. Straightening my arm and placing my hemiplegic hand on the bathroom countertop made me safer. When my hemiplegic hand didn't stay where I had placed it, I knew I was swaying away from vertical during a task. This early feedback told me I needed to correct my posture before I fell. If you feel insecure about working in standing during your early recovery, being able to straighten your hemiplegic arm and place your hand on a surface may make you safer too.

Leaning on an extended arm helped me get rid of the bad habit of standing up with most of my weight on my sound leg. I place my hemiplegic hand on my hemiplegic thigh and stand up by straightening my elbow. This tactile cue reminds me to stand up symmetrically so my sound leg doesn't tire so quickly because it is doing most of the work. Leaning on my extended hemiplegic arm in this way helps me get on and off the **toilet** when I'm tired **at night** and not fully awake in the morning.

After my **balance** improved, it was safe for me to lean down in standing to straighten the bed linen by placing my hand on the nightstand and leaning on my extended hemiplegic arm. Leaning on an extended arm makes me more stable and is less tiring for my back. However, bending over in standing to lean on your extended hemiplegic arm may not be safe for you. Have your OT evaluate if leaning on an extended hemiplegic arm increases or decreases your safety during tasks that are meaningful to you.

While I was amazed at what a hemiplegic arm can do, I was still worried about my hemiplegic hand because hand recovery is often poor. As a therapist, I knew from experience that many stroke survivors get better return in their leg than they do in their hand.

Why Recovery is Harder for the Hand

Recovery of the hand is influenced by two factors that promote disuse even when you make motor gains. The first factor is the asymmetrical nature of hand use during ADLs. Walking forces continuous use of both legs, but forced use of the hemiplegic hand is often intermittent during ADLs. For example, filling and emptying a clothes dryer can be done one-handed except for the ten seconds when you need both hands to clean the lint trap after each load. The first time stroke survivors learn about the limitations of one-handed techniques may be when we go home and are left alone. When we no longer have a small army of hospital staff to retrieve and prepare task materials, we are likely to experience task disruption. Not being able to get the cap off the milk container may mean you can't prepare breakfast if your spouse is in the shower or you decide to sleep in while a caregiver runs errands. Are you relying too much on one-handed techniques that can leave you stranded? Repeatedly not being able to finish what you start can lead to learned helplessness.

The second factor that promotes disuse of the hemiplegic hand is the ease with which caregivers do fine-motor tasks. Caregivers may be intimidated by lifting a body, but it's hard to watch a loved one struggle when it is so easy for a caregiver to reach over and zip up your coat. It is hard to prevent disuse when everyone sees that you don't know how to use early hand movement. Once you and the people who take care of you silently negotiate the contract that therapists call disuse, it is hard to change a habit that is a part of how you and your family interact every day. Fortunately, innovations like constraint-induced therapy and the next generation of electrical stimulation devices have changed this poor outcome for the hand.

Good News from Constraint-Induced Therapy

A psychologist got the idea to restrain the sound hand with a sling or hand splint for three to six hours a day. This physical restraint forces stroke survivors to use their hemiplegic hand. However, constraint-induced therapy doesn't just restrain the sound arm and hope for the best. While the sound hand is constrained, therapists have the hemiplegic hand do repetitive tasks that range from easy tasks, like stacking plastic cones, to more difficult tasks, like screwing nuts and bolts together.

Taub and his associates (1993) found that four stroke survivors who had some movement in their wrist and fingers made new motor gains even though they'd had a stroke from one to eighteen *years* earlier. Motor gains included a stronger, faster grasp and an arm that could move through a greater range of active movement. Other researchers followed suit and found similar results. See the short list of references at the end of this chapter. The news that adults who participate in constraint-induced therapy regain hand use years after their stroke is encouraging. A popular belief in the rehabilitation community is that the motor return you get in the first six to twelve months is pretty much it. Research on constraint-induced therapy has proven that this is not always true.

Despite these encouraging results, I didn't participate in constraint therapy. First, I live alone and have to do self-care, prepare meals, do laundry, clean my house, and shop so I can't have my sound hand restrained for extended periods. Second, I didn't have any active movement in my hemiplegic wrist and fingers two months after my stroke. Stroke survivors who didn't have some wrist and finger movement were excluded from the constraint studies. Fortunately, new expectations also produced a wave of new technology for the hemiplegic hand. One such device called NeuroMove gave me active hand movement and will be discussed in the next section. Living alone is frustrating because one-handed techniques eventually lead to failure when there is no one there to rescue you. Living alone produced my own version of forced use of the hemiplegic hand.

Electrical Stimulation for the Hemiplegic Hand

I asked Dr. Terry who oversaw my inpatient rehabilitation to prescribe NeuroMove because I didn't have any movement in my hemiplegic hand when I went home. I had never heard of this device when I was a therapist, but a friend found it on the Internet. NeuroMove electrically stimulates shoulder, elbow, and wrist muscles when you attach pads to the skin that are connected to the machine with wires. NeuroMove is different from traditional electrical stimulation devices that stimulate muscles at regular intervals regardless of whether or not you are trying to move. NeuroMove doesn't let you sit there and wait for it to do the work. It stimulates your muscles only when the biofeedback component tells the machine you are trying to initiate a movement. NeuroMove is also different because the machine gives verbal commands that tell the user what to do at each step.

Here is one example of how NeuroMove works. When you cannot see your wrist move, you can watch a line on the monitor that shows your muscle activity as soon you start thinking about moving. Watching that line creep higher and higher as your muscle activity increases encourages you to try harder. As soon as the line that tracks your muscle activity rises above the horizontal threshold set by the machine, you get a few seconds of electric stimulation and are rewarded with a visible movement. If you get frustrated because you can't get above the threshold set by the machine, you can lower the threshold until you can succeed. After a few successes, the machine automatically raises the threshold line slightly. Although I never lost awareness of what position my joints were in when other people moved them, I had no clue about where the muscles that controlled my wrist and hand were located. The biofeedback component helped me find muscles I didn't know I still had.

The biofeedback component is helpful in another way. I was flabbergasted to learn that my wrist muscles were working all the time, even when my arm was hanging straight down at my side. The only way I could get my wrist muscles to relax was to rest my forearm on a table and completely empty my mind. No wonder my muscles fatigued so quickly in therapy. I had lost the ability to make my muscles relax when my therapist said "rest for a while." Therapists have known for decades that stroke survivors have trouble turning off a muscle after they recruit it. NeuroMove won't administer the next electrical stimulation until the biofeedback component says you have completely relaxed the muscle you just used.

The good news is that NeuroMove can teach you to initiate voluntary movement. It is affordable and practical. I paid a rental fee of $100 a month in 2004. I was able to place the reusable sticky pads on my hemiplegic forearm and wrist one-handed. Leave the pads attached to the wires so you only have to plug the wires into the machine at the beginning of each treatment session. I put the pads in a zip-lock bag and left the wires hanging out of the opening. You can learn more about NeuroMove by going to www.neuromove.com and by reading the two articles listed at the end of this chapter.

The bad news is that researchers haven't proven that NeuroMove has a positive impact on hemiplegic hand use during ADLs. Page and Levine concluded that subjects who used NeuroMove "showed no functional changes" (p. 29, 2006). Another electrical stimulation device called Bioness, which costs $6,200, has shown inconsistent results. One study showed that twenty-nine subjects were able to use their hemiplegic hand during ADLs while wearing the Bioness, but this effect disappeared when they took the device off (Alon, McBride, & Ring, 2002). In a second study, one stroke survivor used the Bioness as part of a rigorous OT treatment program (Hill-Hermann et al., 2008). After three weeks of treatment, she reported increased use of her hemiplegic hand during ADL tasks when she wasn't wearing the Bioness. Researchers aren't going to find positive functional change after electrical stimulation as long as they use tests that don't measure what the hemiplegic hand does during ADL tasks. Stroke survivors need a functional test for the hemiplegic hand that justifies continued treatment of the hemiplegic hand and compels our insurance companies to pay for it.

Evaluation of the Hemiplegic Hand is Outdated

Since the 1960s, therapists have evaluated the hemiplegic hand by asking clients to pick up and put down objects, like a tennis ball. Assessing grasp and release outside of a useful context does not tell us if the ability to pick up and put down objects actually increases independence during ADLs. Other test items typically ask clients to manipulate objects during quasi-functional tasks, like scooping up beans with a spoon and putting them in a small container, putting blocks in a box, and putting marbles on top of a box. Quasi-functional tasks use common objects that make them appear functional, but what does success or failure on tasks like these tell us about the ability to perform authentic ADL tasks? Using a spoon to drop a bean into a container does not mean you can keep the spoon level as you take it to your mouth. Placing small round objects on top of a box doesn't mean you can push thin flat buttons through buttonholes. The problem with using quasi-functional tasks to predict functional performance is that they are simpler than real ADL tasks.

Making quasi-functional tasks simple does not give them a good basement. A test with a good basement shows progress across several beginning levels of skill rather than judging you on a single skill. Stroke survivors often fail when asked to pick up objects with their hemiplegic hand because this task is not testing a beginning level skill. Even normal infants practice easier versions of hand use first, like holding on to a toy that is placed in their hand. Adults can practice early hand use without resorting to infantile activities. An adult task that requires early hand use is using the sound hand to place a deodorant bottle in the hemiplegic hand so it can hold the bottle as the sound hand removes the cap.

Another reason quasi-functional hand tests don't have a good basement is that they don't allow therapists to provide assistance when clients fail fine-motor test items. Therapists provide physical assistance that varies from minimal to maximal when they lift clients out of a wheelchair. Assistance that requires dozens of pounds to differentiate between levels doesn't help therapists document progress during fine-motor tasks. It is also difficult to provide smooth, accurate assistance during fine-motor tasks. If you have ever tried to help a toddler scoop up food with a spoon by placing your hand over the toddler's hand you know what I mean. There is a simple solution. If a task is too difficult, you can modify it to make it easier, like wrapping **non-slip shelf liner** around the deodorant bottle to help a client hold on to it. Clients are not used to being given a second chance to succeed in a modified way, but a test with a good basement tries to discover what clients can do instead of documenting what they cannot do. Modifying a functional task is a more age-appropriate way to grade down task difficulty than asking adults to put blocks in a box.

Current functional tests have difficulty proving that the hemiplegic hand can improve because these tests also lack good basements for fine-motor ADL tasks. For example, self-feeding is the easiest task on the Functional Independence Measure (FIM) (Fischer, 1993). Since many stroke survivors never regain the ability to manage a spoon with their hemiplegic hand, it is easy to see why the FIM rarely shows that a hemiplegic hand can be functional. The Arm Motor Ability Test (AMAT) is a more recent attempt to assess hemiplegic hand use during ADLs. It does not have a good basement either. The majority of AMAT test items require isolated finger control or wrist and forearm mobility. High-level AMAT items include tying shoes and turning a doorknob. Even opening a door is difficult because you have to rotate the forearm while keeping your hand relaxed and extending your elbow. Turning your hand palm up isn't functional if your hand gets stuck on the doorknob because your hand closes into a fist. So it is not surprising that Chae and his associates (2003) concluded that the AMAT underestimates arm control in people with more severe strokes.

Current functional tests are designed for stroke survivors who have substantial fine-motor recovery while people with more severe strokes are the target group for new technology, like NeuroMove. This mismatch can have serious repercussions. Clients may jump to conclusions when they are not given functional tests they can pass. I know a stroke survivor who threw his technology in the closet when he lost hope. When the only objects stroke survivors are handed are cones, beanbags, balls, and blocks, it's hard to sustain our commitment to a rigorous hand therapy program. We need to see early functional progress that begins to change our life at home. We need more than the implied promise that "your hand will be useful someday."

After my stroke I created the Test of Early Bilateral Hand Use (TEBHU) so clients could get credit for using their hemiplegic hand during ADLs. Eleven stroke survivors who participated in field trials of the TEBHU illustrate the kind of movement you need to make your hemiplegic hand functional. Adults who were *limited to* making a partial fist and placing their hemiplegic hand on their thigh without flinging it there were not recruited (TEBHU Level 1). Adults who could open their hemiplegic hand one to two inches without help from the sound hand could do bimanual ADLs at TEBHU Level 2. Adults who could reach out and grab an object with their hemiplegic hand could do bimanual ADLs at Levels 3 and 4. Adults who had some isolated movement of individual fingers could do bimanual ADLs at Level 5. If you can do any of the arm and hand movements described above, think about trying the following TEBHU strategies. They may help you increase your independence during fine-motor ADL tasks.

Making the Hemiplegic Hand Functional

Strategies able-bodied people never use. Able-bodied people use their fingers to hold down an object while they manipulate it, like pressing their index finger next to the dotted line as they tear a return stub from a bill. What stroke survivors may have to do instead is use their whole hand, either open or fisted, to trap an object (TEBHU Level 1). You may think that holding objects still by pressing down on them with your hemiplegic hand isn't true hand function, but I hope I can change your mind.

It's true that trapping an object with your whole hand isn't as elegant as extending your index finger to hold down a ribbon while you tie a bow. Yet the feeling of empowerment that comes from being able to trap objects can be profound. Here is an example of what I mean. My hand wasn't heavy enough to hold down a wad of **toilet paper** I placed on my thigh so I could tear it. Jerking quickly doesn't always work, especially if the roll is light when it's almost empty. It's frustrating when the roll unwinds and you have to slowly rewind it with one hand. This happened to me again and again. I think I've rewound a mile of toilet paper. Well, maybe not a mile, but in four months I rewound a lot of toilet paper. If you have ever had a toddler or a kitten who thinks it is fun to unroll toilet paper until there is a pool of paper on the floor then you know how frustrated I felt. Here is a partial list of the objects I am really glad to be able to trap (TERHU Level 1). *Note.* SH = sound hand and HH = hemiplegic hand.

Level 1: Trapping Objects

- While sitting on a **shower chair**, HH traps the head of the shower hose against the lower abdomen while the SH rinses the crotch.
- To keep from dumping lots of **shampoo** on head while holding the bottle overhead, HH traps an oval-shaped shampoo bottle on thigh as the SH tilts the bottle down and catches the shampoo.
- To open a box of cereal, the hand, wrist, and part of the forearm of the hemiplegic arm trap the box against stomach so the SH can open the lid.
- To hold a checkbook open, place a stapler on one edge of the checkbook and the HH on the other edge so the SH can make an entry.
- To get money out of a wallet, rest HH and hemiplegic wrist against stomach to support an opened wallet as the SH takes money out.
- SH opens newspaper stand and HH traps the door open so it won't slam on SH as it retrieves a paper.

A second strategy able-bodied people never use is to pick up a small object with their non-dominant hand and transfer it to the dominant hand before they use the object. However, stroke survivors may initially have to pick up an object with the sound hand and place it in the hemiplegic hand. After the hemiplegic hand receives an object, the TEBHU allows a client to hold the object close to the body, prop the object against the hip or stomach, or rest the object on the table or lap as long as the hemiplegic hand doesn't let go. Early hand use is more likely if you don't have to take the full weight of an object or lift your arm far away from your body. The Neurodevelopmental Treatment approach has taught OTs to think that good arm control has to come *before* hand use, but this is not always true. PTs put a brace on the ankle and walk clients long before they have good hip and knee control. Why defer early hand use when modified tasks can make do with emerging arm and hand control?

Transferring objects from hand to hand also facilitates early release. Even before active finger extension is visible, your hemiplegic hand may be able to relax enough to slide off of an object as your sound hand takes it. If you have trouble opening your hand to receive or let go of an object, try a hand-above-hand transfer. At lap height, hold your palm-down hemiplegic hand above your palm-up sound hand. This hand-above-hand position may allow you to drop your hemiplegic hand. A bent wrist position may partially straighten your fingers so your hemiplegic hand can open enough to take or let go of an object.

The first time I spontaneously used my hemiplegic hand after using NeuroMove, I didn't realize what I had done until it was over. Without thinking, my sound hand had put a videotape cover in my hemiplegic hand and then slid the videotape inside. Seeing that videotape in its cover stopped me in my tracks. I stared at the videotape and tried again and succeeded. My brain had grown a new connection to an old memory I thought I had lost forever.

Here are two partial lists of functional tasks that can be done when your sound hand picks up an object and places it in the hemiplegic hand, which holds the object close to the body. *Note*: SH = sound hand and HH = hemiplegic hand. Some stroke survivors can hold objects that are placed between their palm and thumb (TEBHU Level 2a). Some stroke survivors can also hold objects that are placed between their fingertips and thumb (TEBHU Level 2b).

Level 2a: Object Between Palm and Thumb

- While sitting on a **shower chair**, SH places the head of shower hose in HH, which holds the nozzle still as the SH rinses the crotch.
- SH places a deodorant bottle in the HH so SH can remove the cap (Ban roll-on has an hour-glass shape that is easy to hold on to).
- SH places a full tube of toothpaste in the HH, which rests the end of the tube on the hip as it holds the toothpaste so the SH can take off the cap.
- In sitting, SH places hair dryer in the HH. My HH holds the hair dryer as I lean forward to rest my hemiplegic forearm on my thigh (leaning over may not be safe for you). SH lifts and fluffs hair.
- SH places **cane** in the HH, which holds cane at side of body as SH closes bathroom door.
- SH places a cordless phone in HH, which holds it at side of body while walking with a **cane** to sit down to have a conversation on the couch or take notes while sitting at a table.

Level 2b: Object Between Fingertips and Thumb

- SH puts a teabag between thumb and fingertips of HH, which hold bag as SH pulls the string from the bag.
- SH puts envelope between thumb and fingertips of HH, which hold the envelope as SH removes a bill or card (fold **non-slip shelf liner** over envelope if needed).
- SH places the bottom flap of a zip-lock sandwich bag between the thumb and fingertips of HH, which hold flap still as SH grasps the top flap and pulls it upwards to open the bag.

If you feel helpless during fine-motor tasks, your family senses this and does things for you without being asked. If you acquire Level 1 or 2 skills, it can change everyone's perception of your hemiplegic hand. When everyone understands the value of small arm and hand movements, positive expectations can produce positive outcomes.

Skills able-bodied people take for granted. In addition to using strategies that able-bodied people never use, stroke survivors can use manual skills able-bodied people overlook. Able-bodied people don't pay attention to simple hand movements that don't require precise finger control, such as static grasp. Static grasp is the ability to close the hand around an object and hold on to it. While current hand evaluations assess static grasp, they ignore its functional significance. Reaching out and holding an object still is so effortless for able-bodied people that this simple skill *slips below their level of awareness.* Able-bodied people who take the cap off a milk container don't pay attention to the hand holding the container to keep it still. They don't pay attention to the hand holding the cord out of the way while they vacuum. See a partial list of TEBHU Level 3 tasks listed below. *Note:* Some tasks require the two hands to function at different levels. SH = sound hand and HH = hemiplegic hand.

Level 3: Reaching Out to Hold an Object

- HH reaches out to hold a yogurt container (Level 3) as the SH pulls the top open and uses a spoon to scrape the last of the yogurt from the bottom of the container (Level 5).
- HH reaches out to hold a pot handle to keep it completely still (Level 3) so the pot won't tip and spill hot food or slide off the burner as SH stirs the contents with a spoon (Level 4).
- HH holds lint trap of a dryer away from body (Level 3) as SH scoops out lint (Level 4).
- HH reaches out to hold a dough scraper as the SH pushes diced garlic/onions onto the scraper. Both hands hold the scraper as they lift it to dump the food in a container or pot.
- HH reaches out to grab the handle of a food processor container and press the container against stomach (Level 3) as the SH scoops out food sticking to sides (Level 4).
- Both hands reach out and hold the grab bar of a **shopping cart** to propel and steer it around a store.
- Church: Both arms reach out to the side so your hands can grasp hands of people on either side of you.

- To reposition the driver's seat after a mechanic works on your car: Place HH on steering wheel; SH presses the release bar while HH on the steering wheel pulls the seat forward.

In addition to holding objects still, static grasp is functional in a second way that able-bodied people don't pay attention to. After your hand grasps an object, many objects are manipulated with the wrist and forearm, like turning a page. Able-bodied people think about wrist and forearm movements that change the position of the hand during difficult tasks, like swinging a golf club. However, they make these adjustments automatically and effortlessly during simple ADLs. Yet a stroke survivor whose wrist and forearm are tight or limp is painfully aware of how many objects are manipulated with wrist and forearm mobility. See a partial list of TEBHU Level 4 tasks below. *Note*: Some equipment dictates what each hand does (e.g., does the refrigerator door open to the left or right?). Some tasks require the two hands to function at different levels. SH = sound hand and HH = hemiplegic hand. Level 4 tasks can be bilateral (4a) or unilateral (4b).

Level 4a: Bilateral Wrist/Forearm Mobility

- To pull up your pants, both hands grab the waistband and your wrists gradually bend as you pull the pants up to your waist.
- Wrist of one hand continuously bends as it pulls the refrigerator door open and wrist of other hand continuously adjusts to keep the food level while placing it on a shelf.
- SH holds the handle of a pot (Level 3) while the HH uses a wooden spoon to stir the contents of the pot (Level 4).
- Buckling a lap-type seat belt: One hand holds the part that receives tab (Level 3) as wrist and forearm of other hand adjust continuously as they bring belt across lap (Level 4).
- Zipping a coat: As SH holds bottom of coat, HH pulls zipper to the top of coat (This is Level 4 because the wrist must gradually bend more and more without the hand opening and dropping the tab.)

Level 4b: Unilateral Wrist/Forearm Mobility
- Pick up telephone and turn it as you take it to your ear.
- Comb or brush your hair.
- Turn a key in the lock and turn doorknob to open door.
- Drink from a glass, continuously adjusting the wrist and forearm to keep from spilling.
- Scoop up food with a spoon and continuously adjust the wrist and forearm to keep the spoon level so food will not spill as you take it to your mouth.

Try two-handed ADLs. On current ADL evaluations, test items that target the hemiplegic hand are often unilateral, like using a spoon (TEBHU Level 4b). When the dominant hand is affected, two-handed tasks are better at detecting functional recovery than one-handed tasks. You get credit for using your hemiplegic hand as the dominant hand during easy tasks and continue to get credit for using it as the assistive hand when task difficulty increases. Your OT can analyze the tasks that made your hemiplegic hand switch roles and design a program that targets the skills it needs to be a fully dominant hand again. Two-handed test items are especially useful when the non-dominant hand is affected. Two-handed tasks allow the non-dominant hand to perform the familiar role of being an assistive hand. Evaluating a non-dominant hand by asking it to do one-handed tasks *it never did* when you were well makes it easy to overlook early recovery. Ask to be evaluated with some two-handed ADL tasks.

You don't have to choose between using both hands or using the hemiplegic hand alone. Therapy sessions and home programs that use one-handed tasks are an excellent way to retrain the hemiplegic hand. Yet you don't have to defer hand use during ADLs until your hemiplegic hand is good enough to manipulate objects by itself. Try two-handed ADLs instead of waiting for your hemiplegic hand to get better. A few minutes of exercise each day cannot overcome twelve hours of disuse. As soon as you get a little motor return, you either use it or lose it!

Use task modification. Task modification has been used for a long time to compensate for a lack of hand recovery, like using a rocker knife to cut food one-handed. **Task modification** can also be used to increase hand use, like propping the end of a full tube of toothpaste on your hip while your sound hand removes the cap. Give yourself permission to discover your own way to modify ADL tasks. Feel free to ignore the task modifications I've included in Levels 1-4 tasks if you don't need them. *Note*: SH = sound hand and HH = hemiplegic hand.

Suggested Task Modifications
- Use your SH to place an object in HH and retrieve it.
- Begin by grasping objects you can hold close to your body, like a cane.
- If you have trouble holding an object, prop it against your stomach or hip or rest it on your lap or the table without letting go. Propping reduces the amount of weight your hemiplegic hand initially has to hold.
- Wrap **non-slip shelf liner** around objects or place it under objects to create friction to help you hold on to the object.
- Stand to do tasks you normally do seated so you don't have to lift your arm as high, like standing to open envelopes or staple sheets of a bill together.
- If you have trouble *opening* your HH to grasp an object, relax your fingers by bending your wrist. Press the back of your HH against a piece of furniture if needed.
- If you have trouble *closing* your HH on an object, put the object down and practice the grasp without the object in your HH. Rehearsal may increase muscle tone.

Many ADL tasks are possible at each level. Your hemiplegic hand can help you manipulate up to *seventy-six* ADL objects before it can pick up objects and set them down. This list includes opening twenty-five objects. People who provide set-up assistance are robbing stroke survivors of many opportunities for early hand use. If you recover wrist and forearm mobility, your hemiplegic hand can help you manipulate up to *twenty-eight* ADL objects. I am not padding the number by counting woodworking tools, like a hammer. I hope the partial lists for Levels 1-4 give you an idea of what you might be able to do with your hemiplegic hand. Regaining simple manual skills is worth it. These skills can be used again and again in different contexts, just as walking allows you to get to the bed, toilet, kitchen table, couch, and car. I have plateaued at Level 3 with a few Level 4 skills, but the TEBHU strategies have made me independent in *eighty* two-handed fine-motor ADL tasks at home and in the community.

Finding the Ceiling

The ceiling for hand use during ADLs includes Level 5 tasks on the TEBHU. These tasks require individual fingers to conform to the shape and size of different tools, like a knife. Different fingers doing different movements, like extending the index finger over the top of a knife while the thumb and middle finger grasp the opposite sides of the handle, achieve this contouring effect. You need strength to maintain that contour against resistance, like cutting through food, keeping tension on shoelaces as you tie a bow, and pushing a button through a buttonhole. Level 5 tasks are the golden standard for hand use during ADLs so it is easy to see why some people feel pessimistic about functional recovery in the hemiplegic hand. Yet giving up because you can't do Level 5 tasks doesn't make sense to me. Are your expectations for your hemiplegic hand helping you or holding you back?

The ceiling for hand use during ADLs also includes learning to **multitask**. After my stroke, I used to watch the opening sequence of *Mister Rogers' Neighborhood* with awe and envy. Mister Rogers would waltz down the stairs, take off his jacket, turn to face the closet, open the door, put his jacket on a hanger, and don and zip his sweater while simultaneously singing, smiling, and whipping his head around to make eye contact with the camera. I am at the other end of the continuum. The effort to keep my hemiplegic hand closed is so intense at first that I can't think about anything else. If I divert my attention to my sound hand, my hemiplegic hand opens involuntarily as though I'm holding a hot rock. Even if I give myself strict instructions to hold on to an object, my hemiplegic hand opens against my will the moment my attention is diverted.

Here are two examples of how **multitasking** currently affects my hand function. First, I can hold the tube of mascara with my hemiplegic hand, but it drops the tube as soon as I grab the wand with my sound hand to apply the mascara. A second example is talking and using my hemiplegic hand at the same time. People think my hemiplegic hand is useless when they see it lying motionless on my lap while I talk to them. What people perceive as a lack of voluntary hand movement is really my inability to multitask.

I learned to multitask while moving my hemiplegic leg, so I haven't given up hope. This success helped me accept that failure is a necessary part of regaining motor control. If I regain the ability to hold an object and practice the task over and over, I have succeeded at multitasking while using my hand. For example, I can use both hands to zip up my coat and say goodbye to people at the same time. Small triumphs like this make my day.

If your hemiplegic hand recovers enough to be your dominant hand, you may have less difficulty with multitasking than I do because you won't have to divide your attention in an unnatural way. If you have ever hit your finger while hammering a nail you learned to pay closer attention to the dominant hand controlling the hammer. When an OT gives your dominant hand a one-handed task to perform, that therapeutic task replicates the intense concentration people often give their dominant hand during functional tasks.

Stroke survivors who use their hemiplegic hand as an assistive hand don't have this luxury. We concentrate intensely on our hemiplegic hand during one-handed tasks, but initially have to divide our attention during two-handed tasks. We focus on our sound hand to make sure it's working with precision and then switch our focus to the assistive hemiplegic hand when it doesn't cooperate. Learning to use a hemiplegic hand as an assistive hand takes patience. The initial results when you try to transfer what you've learned to a two-handed task can be discouraging. Using one hand at a time is simple by comparison.

If you don't recover the ability to multitask while using your hemiplegic hand, you have to make choices. Do you want to keep talking or are you willing to create a lull in the conversation while you concentrate on using your hemiplegic hand? Do you want to keep walking or do you want to stop and use your hemiplegic hand? At the mall, I step out of the stream of traffic and stand next to a wall to zip my winter coat. There is no right answer; it's a matter of what is important to you at the moment. A hemiplegic hand has a better chance of succeeding if you initially reduce the number of demands a situation requires. When I ask my hemiplegic hand to do something difficult, I cheat by making another part of the task easier. If your hemiplegic hand is struggling, ask yourself if all the other things you are doing at the same time are really necessary.

The Bottom Line

I don't mean to imply that retraining the hemiplegic hand is easy. Poor sensation, painful joints, and tight or floppy muscles are just some of the deficits that create genuine roadblocks to recovery. For example, the more times I closed my hand on objects after I unplugged the NeuroMove machine, the tighter my hand got. By dinnertime I couldn't open my hemiplegic hand without help from my sound hand. It took a talented OT named Melissa to help me regain use of my hand. After an intense out-patient program, she gave me a home program to keep my progress going. My hand still gets tight so I use a SaeboFlex splint that has springs to help me open my hand (www.saebo.com). I wear the splint while I pick up and let go of 125 balls each day. The first twenty-five repetitions just work out the stiffness. Think about how many times you put weight on your hemiplegic leg before you left the hospital. Repeated forced use of the hemiplegic leg during walking shows us that retraining the brain takes *hundreds* of repetitions.

Your success will also depend on helping your family understand what they can do to support your recovery. To prevent hurt feelings, talk to your caregivers about the fine-motor tasks you want to do yourself and the tasks you prefer that other people do for you. Renegotiate every time your hand makes progress. See if combining traditional therapy, innovative treatments, a functional hand evaluation with a good basement, and communication with caregivers gives you a better outcome.

Regaining hand function is an emotional roller coaster that takes many twists and turns. One thing that surprised me about hand recovery was learning I had been spoiled by a world that catered to my needs when I was right-handed. Now that my sound left hand is my dominant hand, I have to deal with a car that has the ignition on the right side, credit cards that have to be swiped on the right side of many machines, and a camera with a button on the right side that controls the shutter. I wonder if people who are born left-handed are more aware of the simple things hands do because they are forced to think about hand use all their lives. The left-handed guy who fixes my computer doesn't go around messing up everyone's computer layout by moving their mouse pad to the left side.

Another thing that surprised me is how little my hand can do when I'm given a verbal instruction to move it. Yet if I slap an object in my hemiplegic hand, it often responds without my thinking about it. For instance, there weren't enough chairs around the table one Thanksgiving so my friend got out some stools. Someone handed me a stool. Both of my hands reached out and grasped the stool and set it down. I didn't realize what I had done until it was over. I am lucky because this has happened again and again. Forced use with *familiar* objects helped my brain grow new connections to old motor memories. You may be able to follow verbal commands to do hand movements, but in the final analysis hand use is a *visual*-motor skill. I am still astonished by the power familiar functional objects have to elicit unexpected recovery.

The last thing that surprised me was learning how much of my self-worth is tied up in my hands. It is wonderful to be able to walk again, but I want to be the master of my world when I get where I am going. I am grateful to have enough function in my hemiplegic hand to be able to stay in my own home. This is a huge payoff for all my hard work. Therapists call my hemiplegic hand a "functional assist." I call it my blessed hand.

Annotated Bibliography

Alon, G, McBride, K., & Ring, H. (2002). Improving selected hand functions using a noninvasive neuroprosthesis in persons with chronic stroke. *Journal of Stroke & Cerebrovascular Diseases, 11*

(2), 99-105. An early study of the Bioness device when it was called the Handmaster.

Chae, J., Labatia, I., & Yang, G. (2003). Upper limb motor function in hemiparesis: Concurrent validity of the Arm Motor Ability Test. *American Journal of Physical Medicine, 82*(1), 1-8. The AMAT tests hemiplegic hand use during ADLs, but it does not have a good basement.

Fisher, W.P. (1993). Measurement-related problems in functional assessment. *American Journal of Occupational Therapy, 47* (4), 331-338. A critique of self-care evaluations.

Gillot, A., Holder-Walls, A., Kurtz, J., & Varley, N. (2003). Perceptions and experiences of two survivors of stroke who participated in constraint-induced movement therapy home programs. *American Journal of Occupational Therapy, 57* (2), 168-176. An easy to understand article that clearly describes what happened to two clients who participated in constraint therapy.

Hill-Hermann, V., Strasser, A., Albers, B., Scholield, K., Dunning, K., Levine. P., & Page, S. (2008). Task-specific, patient-driven neuroprosthesis training in chronic stroke: Results from a 3-week clinical study. *American Journal of Occupational Therapy, 62*(4), 466-472. One client's experience with an electrical stimulation device called Bioness.

Kraft, G., Fitts, S., & Hammond, M. (1992). Techniques to improve function of the arm and hand in chronic hemiplegia. *Archives of Physical Medicine and Rehabilitation, 73*, 220-227. A study of an early version of NeuroMove when it was called AutoMove.

Page, S., & Levine, P. (2006). Back from the brink: Electromyography-triggered stimulation combined with modified constraint-induced movement therapy in chronic stroke. *Archives of Physical Medicine and Rehabilitation, 87*, 27-31. Combining NeuroMove and constraint therapy.

Page, S., Levine, P., & Hill, V. (2007). Mental practice as a gateway to modified constraint-induced movement therapy: A promising combination to improve function. *American Journal of Occupational Therapy, 61* (3), 321-327.

Taub, E., Miller, N., Novack, T., Cook, E., Fleming, W., Nepomuceno,

C., Connell, J., & Crago, J. (1993). Technique to improve chronic motor deficit after stroke. *Archives of Physical Medicine and Rehabilitation, 74*, 347-354. An early study of constraint-induced therapy.

More articles are listed at the end of each article above.

CHAPTER 4

BASIC SELF-CARE

I regained independence in self-care, not because I wanted to be a model patient, but because I don't have anyone at home to tell "honey, do this." I'm divorced and wasn't able to have children. My parents are dead. My surviving siblings live in Illinois and California while I live in New Jersey. I thought I could go to assisted living before going home to live alone. Then I discovered the assisted-living facility near my home doesn't accept people who can't toilet themselves. This news lit a fire under me!

Another reason for regaining my independence surprised me. It was irritating to have to wait ten minutes for someone to answer my call button when I was in the hospital. When my hospital stay dragged on for two months, waiting really got old. It's maddening when you have to wait for everything. Being able to dress myself meant I no longer had to watch my breakfast get cold while I waited for an aide to come back to finish dressing me and put the breakfast tray in front of me. Being able to get off the toilet independently meant I no longer had to freeze as I sat on the toilet wearing a skimpy hospital gown while I waited for an aide to come back to transfer me. When you are waiting, one minute can seem like fifteen unless you go mentally numb. It was scary to know that it took just two months to turn me into Forrest Gump – the guy who puts his son on the school bus, tells him "I'll be right here," and sits down to stare blankly into space all day.

Gadgets versus What You Carry with You

Before I go into specifics, I want to talk about four general strategies that promote independence. While gadgets look like a quick fix, they are the last solution I turn to. The first compensatory strategy I use is changing my body **position**. If you are struggling with a task, it helps to straighten up. For instance, if you are having trouble straightening a wet towel on a towel rack, it helps to face the wall instead of reaching while your torso is twisted. Sometimes it helps to change your position more drastically, like standing when you would

58

normally sit. For instance, you may have better leverage when you stand up to staple credit card bills together to keep them in order. Changing your body position is quick and may be all you need to do to succeed.

The second compensatory strategy I turn to is called in-hand manipulation, which means using some fingers to hold an object while other fingers of the same hand manipulate the object. A clarinetist uses some fingers to hold the clarinet and other fingers to cover the holes. An everyday example is putting money in a vending machine. We hold the coins in our palm and then use our fingers to slide the coins out to our fingertips to put the coins in the slot without ever using the other hand. The best part of in-hand manipulation is that we always have our fingers and thumbs with us. I recommend using it whenever you can.

I call the third compensatory strategy the **"backwards rule."** I can't describe the general characteristics of this strategy because I don't see the common thread that makes it so successful. For example, people usually clean their eyeglasses by bringing a cloth to their glasses, but it is easier for one-handed people to bring their eyeglasses to the cloth. Lay a cloth on the table, lay your eyeglasses on top of the cloth, and pick up a corner or an edge of the cloth to wipe each lens. To pump hand lotion from a bottle with one hand, turn the pump away from you. If you bend all four fingers while you press on the pump, you can catch the liquid in your cupped fingers as your palm presses down on the plunger. Look for other examples of the backwards rule throughout the book. When I am struggling with a task, I try doing it backwards.

Of course, some problems can be solved only with an adaptive device, which is equipment that performs some manual function you cannot do. A nail clipper mounted on a suction-cup base allows you to press down on the lever arm of the clipper with your hemiplegic hand (opened or closed) to trim the nails on your sound hand. However, using a gadget is the last strategy I turn to because it takes precious energy to get up and retrieve a gadget that is not close by. Except for kitchen gadgets, many adaptive devices require planning ahead so you don't have to interrupt a task to fetch them.

Two adaptive devices that are convenient are clear **Dycem** and non-slip shelf liner. Clear Dycem is flat, thin plastic that is designed to hold paper still while you write. Place large rectangles of it anywhere you sit down to write, like next to the phone to take messages, on the dining table to do crossword puzzles, at your desk to pay bills, and on the table next to the computer to edit a document you've printed out. Women can keep a small piece of clear Dycem in their purse to sign credit card slips. An 8-inch x 2-yard roll costs $30 at www.sammonspreston.com, but the roll can last for a year. I think it's worth every penny. **Non-slip shelf liner** is cheap to replace when it gets dirty. Place small squares around the house to hold objects still, like a pill container, containers of make-up, and dishes on the kitchen counter. Non-slip shelf liner comes in neutral colors that blend with any decorating scheme. Colored Dycem comes in gaudy colors I don't want sitting around my house, clashing with my décor and drawing attention.

Getting Clean Sitting on a Shower Chair

I am going to share some very private information about showering for three reasons. First, the bathroom has a lot of hard surfaces and is a bad place to fall. Second, body odor can negatively affect how people respond to you as a disabled person. Third, taking a shower or bath every day is a pleasure Americans take for granted because they have access to copious amounts of clean water. After you've bathed in the bed and at the sink for two weeks, the sensation of warm, clean water running down your back is luxurious. When an OT watched me shower for the first time, I was self-conscious for about ten seconds. Once the warm water hit my sweaty body and greasy hair, I was in heaven. They could have sold tickets and I wouldn't have cared. The last week I was in the rehab hospital, I got the doctor to write an order for independent showering. I had a big smile on my face every day as I rolled myself down the hall to the shower. It took me two years to lapse back into taking a shower for granted again.

Preparing the bathroom. Installing a grab bar in a shower can be tricky. My shower at home came with a grab bar in the center of the long wall. Unfortunately, the bar is located on my hemiplegic right side where I can't grab it with my sound left hand. My handyman didn't want to create leaks in my fiberglass tub by drilling holes in it. He found a stud along the vertical edge of the tub. My grab bar ended up being vertical, but it is close enough to give me something secure to hold on to. The size of your tub, your height, and the length of your arm will influence where a grab bar needs to be placed in the shower. For safety, the height and location of a shower grab bar must pass two tests. You must be able to (1) hold on to the bar as you sit down on the shower chair and (2) lean forward and grab the bar while sitting before you stand up. Consult with an OT before you place grab bars in your home.

A shower chair and hand-held hose will make you feel safe and are worth every penny. My OT let me try two different shower chairs before she ordered the one that works best for me. Instead of stepping into the shower, you can sit down on the shower chair and swing your legs in afterwards. You will love the notch in the seat of your shower chair because it holds the hand-held hose so you never have to scramble to find it. If you get water in your ears when you rinse your hair, use a hairdresser's trick of keeping the nozzle close to your head. The **Velcro** that came with my shower hose isn't strong enough to hold the nozzle on my wall after I'm through showering. To keep the hand-held nozzle off the floor of the tub when I'm finished, I hang it on a cheap plastic hook designed to hang over a door that I hang on the grab bar inside my tub.

Inexpensive supplies make a shower more enjoyable. Pour shower gel on a nylon-net bath poof so you don't have to chase a slippery bar of soap every time you drop it. A nylon poof is easier to handle one-handed than a washcloth. The nylon poof is easy to grasp, glides easily over your skin, and you don't have to wring it out either. It has a string so you can hang it on a suction-cup hook placed on the shower wall. Bed Bath & Beyond has an assortment of suction-cup devices for hanging bathroom supplies. These devices lose suction about every three or four months and fall off the wall so I wouldn't place anything on them that can break or spill. I love the squeaky clean feeling my shower gel gives me in the summer. However, many shower gels have a lathering agent called sodium sulfate that can dry the skin.

In the winter I use Dove shower gel. It doesn't have sodium sulfate and adds skin softening agents, like glycerin and petroleum jelly. Consider washing your face with lather from your shampoo. My complexion has never looked so good because shampoo lather allows me to wash away the grease along my hairline.

I hated the long-handled bath sponge I got in the rehab hospital. The long handle helps people with hip replacements wash their feet without leaning over. I had to choke up on it like a baseball bat to scrub my back. This made it awkward to use. When I pressed out the excess water, the silky sponge material stayed wet forever. There is no good way to dry it. You can't hang it on a towel rack because the end of the handle is straight. It is too long to fit in a drawer. I stopped counting how many times it fell off my nightstand where I left it to dry and fell off the bathroom sink while I was washing. That long-handled back sponge stayed in the hospital closet when I went home. I love my Buff-Puff back sponge that hangs by its short, curved handle and has a replaceable sponge head that dries quickly. You can order the Buff-Puff from www.drugstore.com.

The last thing I did to prepare the bathroom was put a chair outside the shower. I initially put one there for safety in case I got tired and had to sit down quickly. The chair is a convenient place to keep your towel and bathrobe if your towel rack is too far away from the tub. The chair gives you a place to sit while you undress before you get in the shower and to dry your feet after you get out. However, it's hard to get in and out of the shower if you put the chair in the shower and the outside chair side by side. You need to stand next to your shower chair when you get in and out of the shower. For safety, place the chair outside the tub two or three feet farther back than the shower chair. My friend's bathroom was so tiny there wasn't room to leave a chair out so I used a folding chair. When I moved into my new house, I bought a folding metal chair. The blue metal matches my bathroom décor, which makes me happy.

Procedures once you're in the shower. Standing in a slippery tub requires good **balance**, so it is safer to wash sitting down. Lathering and rinsing your crotch while sitting down is a challenge, but it is possible. At first, I wedged the shower hose in a crease I created by bending my sound hip and used my hemiplegic wrist to press the nozzle against my abdomen so the water ran downward. This freed my sound hand to get into the nooks and crannies. Now I can hold the nozzle with my hemiplegic hand after the sound hand places it there. To clean the rectum, rest the nozzle behind your buttocks on the shower chair, aim the water at the rectum, and push against the hose with your sound knee. You won't actually trap the hose, but the tension you put on the hose helps keep it still. This leaves your sound hand free to wash and rinse.

The one place that is difficult to wash sitting down is my hemiplegic buttock. My sound arm isn't long enough to reach across my body and under the opposite buttock. If you've seen a dog chasing its tail, you'll understand my dilemma. For safety, soap your fanny last so you are not sliding around on a soapy chair. As long as you don't lift your buttocks, your skin stays dry and sticks to the seat.

When you've washed everything except for your buttocks, re-wet the soapy nylon poof and squeeze it behind you so lather runs onto the seat. For safety, hold on to the shower chair with your sound hand and *ever so slightly* slide your hemiplegic buttock forwards and backwards, like a bear rubbing against a tree. This small sliding motion transfers lather from the seat to your hemiplegic buttock. Lathering the sound buttock and rinsing both buttocks is easy if you can raise one buttock at a time without holding on to the shower chair for support. For safety, you may need to hold on to the shower chair with your sound hand while you lift one buttock at a time and let someone else control the shower nozzle to help you rinse.

Drying turned out to be the easiest part. Sitting on the shower chair, drape a towel over one shoulder so half of it hangs down your back to dry it. While the towel absorbs water from your back, use the front half to dry your armpit and arm as best you can. Switch the towel to the other shoulder and repeat. Get out of the shower and don a terry-cloth bathrobe to absorb any remaining moisture on your buttocks, thighs, and upper body. Make the robe easily accessible by hanging it on a cheap plastic hook designed to hang over a door that is hung from a nearby structure, like a towel rack. Sit on the chair next to the tub to dry your feet with a towel. It's easier to put a wet towel on the towel rack if you drape the back half of the towel over your sound shoulder before you push the front half over the rack.

Consider letting your calves air-dry as you brush your teeth, don your underwear, etc. In August when high humidity slows the air-drying process, I lie down on the bed with a dry towel under my legs. Using a terry-cloth bathrobe and resting for a few minutes instead of working up a sweat trying to dry my legs isn't a hard choice for me.

Your bathroom set-up will dictate the equipment and procedures you use to shower, I hope the description of what I do helps you plan ahead. Showering should be associated with pleasure rather than panic. You don't have to choose between feeling safe and feeling clean.

You Can Floss One-Handed

If you don't floss and clean your tongue every day, you won't see what the big deal is. If you do, you know why this task is so important to me. My mouth didn't feel clean for the two months I was in the hospital because I only brushed my teeth. Plackers are disposable, pre-strung floss holders that can be used one-handed. There are several kinds of tongue cleaners that can be used one-handed. Both of these items can be found at drugstores and big discount stores.

Using mouthwash is a little more complicated. It's safe for me to lean forward in sitting to open a child-proof bottle of mouthwash. I put the bottle on the floor between my feet, grab the cap with a generous amount of **non-slip shelf liner** in my sound hand, and push down while I twist the cap. It may not be safe for you to lean forward in sitting. To **prevent a fall**, someone else may need to open the child-proof cap. When you put the cap back on, don't twist it all the way to make it lock. If the bottle is closed loosely, you can open it easily the next time. Some mouthwash probably evaporates, but we're talking about losing pennies. Once you get used to the feeling of a clean mouth, it's hard to go back.

Does Leaning Over Help You Don a Shirt?

OTs routinely teach stroke survivors a procedure designed to get a tight hemiplegic arm through the sleeve of a shirt. Clients are taught to dangle the hemiplegic arm between their knees so gravity will straighten the tight arm before clients put their hand into the sleeve. For a month after my stroke, I couldn't use this procedure. It felt like I was falling whenever I leaned forward in sitting. Was it because I spent so much time lying down and had forgotten where true vertical is? After sitting up during hours of exhausting therapy, I rested every chance I got by lying flat on my back or semi-reclined in bed. Was I afraid because I didn't trust my floppy trunk to stop me once I started to lean forward? Fear is irrational. I could see that I wasn't falling towards the floor but I couldn't reason away my fear.

Even when I had good enough trunk control to **prevent a fall**, it was difficult to see what I was doing if I started dressing by dangling my hemiplegic arm between my knees. It's easier to get your hand in the sleeve opening and part way through the sleeve when the shirt is on your lap. After you have your hand partially through the sleeve, lean forward <u>if it is safe for you</u>, dangle your hemiplegic arm to straighten it, and pull the sleeve up onto your shoulder. Leaning forward also makes it easier to get your head in the neck hole of a pullover top, like a T-shirt or sweater. If you cannot maintain an erect sitting posture when your vision is obstructed by clothing, <u>it's not safe for you</u> to pull the neck hole down over your head while leaning forward. Consider lifting the neck hole over your head when you are sitting upright. It takes more arm strength, but it is safer.

A final step for donning pullover tops, like a T-shirt or sweater, is crucial. After you get the sleeve on your hemiplegic arm and your head through the neck hole, pull the fabric down that is bunched up over your hemiplegic shoulder. Squeeze your shoulder blades together to help the fabric fall down in back if you can. Unless you want to learn what it's like to wiggle out of a straitjacket, do not put your sound arm in its sleeve while the shirt is still bunched up on the other shoulder. Fixing this mistake is aggravating and takes a lot of physical effort. I learned the hard way never to skip this last step when donning a pullover top.

Donning a Short-Leg Brace the Easy Way

Before going into specific procedures, here are a few words about the ankle strap on your brace. Brace makers leave the **Velcro** ankle strap extra long to accommodate different size feet. That means you have to tuck the long tail under the bottom of the brace so it won't bunch up inside your shoe. Once someone crams your brace in your shoe, you can't get at the end of the Velcro strap to open and close it. Consider trimming the ankle strap so you can open and close it after your brace is in your shoe. To cut the Velcro strap to the right length, put your foot in the brace that is already in your shoe, fasten the Velcro strap, and cut it leaving at least a one-inch tail to make it easy to grasp. In four years of walking community distances, my properly cut Velcro strap has never pulled loose. underline For safety, I call my brace man to have the Velcro straps replaced when they get raggedy.

I tried every adapted procedure for putting on a brace that my OT suggested, but failed repeatedly. This was depressing because I couldn't walk safely in bare feet. In sitting, I tried using my sound hand to lift my hemiplegic leg and cross it over my sound leg to bring my hemiplegic foot closer, but my limp hemiplegic leg always slid off. If this classic crossed-leg method doesn't work for you either, here are two alternative ways to **don a shoe**. Both methods involve leaving the brace in the shoe. It is hard even for able-bodied people who have two good hands to put the brace on your leg and cram the brace into a shoe.

When I couldn't keep one leg crossed over the other in sitting, here is what I did. For the first four months, the only way I could put on my leg brace was to sit in the center of the bed with both knees straight in what is called "long-leg sitting." It is not safe to do this procedure if you are sitting close to the edge of the bed. Your legs also have to be flexible enough to get into the long-leg sitting position, so this procedure isn't for everyone.

In long-leg sitting on the bed with the brace in your shoe, slide your toes in the shoe and pull on the brace to get your heel in the shoe. Your toes may point. If this happens, slide your hemiplegic foot up on the bed until your hemiplegic hip and knee are bent like a frog. To push your heel down in the shoe, brace the shoe against your sound leg and push on your hemiplegic knee with your sound hand. The next hurdle is to get the ankle strap through the metal ring on the brace. When your leg is in the frog position, it is flopped open so you can't see the metal ring. Straighten both legs and cross your sound leg on top of your hemiplegic leg. Hook your sound foot over your hemiplegic foot and pull on your toes until they are pointed inwards (i.e., pigeon-toed). Now lean over and push the ankle strap through its ring. If you are not flexible enough to reach down in long-leg sitting to put the strap through the ring, have someone do it for you.

If you lift your hemiplegic leg high enough and keep it still long enough, you may be able to use a second method that involves sitting in a chair to don your shoe and brace. Using this method means you don't have to go back to bed to don a brace. This helps in the community, like after a doctor's examination or when you shop for clothes. While sitting on a chair with your brace in the shoe, lift your shoe by the *tongue*. The weight of the brace will pull the brace down into a horizontal position and make the shoe swing up into a vertical position. Picture a weight pulling a railroad crossing gate up. Once you get your toes in the opening, push your heel down in the shoe by putting your foot on the floor and pushing down on your knee. The brace will act like a shoehorn. Your brace will go on like greased lightning – unless your toes point. Don't panic. Pausing to take a deep breath may relax your muscles so your foot will slide into the shoe. I have mastered this nifty method so I cringe every time a therapist messes me up by taking my brace out of my shoe.

I got lucky the first time I transferred my brace to a new shoe I had bought for the next season. The chair I sit on in my bedroom just happens to be next to a chest of drawers. I accidentally pushed the top of the brace against the chest of drawers. Now I put the toe portion of the brace in the shoe, trap the brace against my trunk with my hemiplegic arm, slide a shoehorn under the heel of the brace with my sound hand, and jam the top of the brace against the chest of drawers and push. Repeated practice helped me get faster and taught me to remember to pull the metal ring out if it gets stuck inside the shoe. See if there is a piece of furniture you can safely push against to get your brace into your shoe while sitting down.

As you can see, there is more than one way to put on your brace. Perhaps my success will help you find a way that works for you. If your hemiplegic ankle buckles when you are barefoot, it is <u>not safe for you</u> and the person helping you if you don't don your brace.

Having the Energy to Worry about Your Hair

In the hospital, I only had enough energy to wash my hair, apply styling gel, comb it, and let it air-dry. When I went home, my hairdresser gave me a curly permanent I could scrunch with my hand and let air-dry. It looked so-so, but I was too exhausted from walking everywhere for the first time in two months to care. Eventually, I had enough energy to do more. A friend recommended a hairdresser who colors my mousy brown hair and gives me a wonderful cut. It's hard to get motivated to go out in public if I'm self-conscious about my hair. Having a good hair day gives me confidence.

Everybody needs to maintain a few hair-care products. Clean your combs and brushes one-handed by using a suction-cup nail brush from www.sammonspreston.com. Wet the suction cups, stick the nailbrush to the wall of your bathroom sink, and pour a little shampoo on it. Wet your comb and hairbrush, drag them repeatedly through the nail brush one at a time, and rinse. Dry the comb by placing it on a towel that is resting on the sink counter and bring the towel to the comb (the **backwards rule**). Small, soft travel containers for shampoo and hair conditioner are easy to handle in the shower, but they run out of product faster than big bottles. To refill them, shove the small travel-size containers into disposable Dixie cups (stack two or three together for strength). Trap the Dixie cups against your stomach with your hemiplegic wrist or grasp them with your hemiplegic hand while you pour in hair product with your sound hand.

Women may want to style their hair. My hair is short so I use a hand-held hair dryer to blow it damp dry, put in Velcro curlers, and let my hair air-dry the rest of the way. I can hold a hair dryer with my hemiplegic hand *if* I sit on a closed toilet seat, rest my forearm on my thigh, and lean over to fluff my wet hair with my sound hand. If you do not have good trunk control, leaning over in sitting is <u>not safe for you.</u>

Consider buying a tall, extendable hair dryer stand at Linens 'n Things or Bed Bath & Beyond that holds a hand-held hair dryer.

I have short hair so I can place **Velcro** curlers one-handed. I found Velcro rollers at upscale drugstores, like CVS, and a beauty supply business that is open to the public. After blowing your hair damp dry, hold the curler with your thumb and middle finger and use your index finger to plow up a section of hair. I stick the curler under this lifted section and turn the curler to pull your hair tight. After combing short hair, keep hairspray out of your ears by putting a cotton ball in your ear.

Elastic Shoelaces Come in What Colors?

For most people, clothes are an important part of their self-image. The only thing that moves me emotionally about clothing is color. So it was unfortunate that I had forgotten elastic shoelaces only come in white, black, and brown. I was appalled when I saw dark brown shoelaces on my tan orthopedic shoes. I was grateful my OT had created a shoe fastening that made me independent, but I was glad I wasn't out in public. When you are invited to your first social event your priority may shift towards appearance. Men are lucky because they can wear dark colored, tie dress shoes that camouflage black or brown elastic laces. When I go to a wedding or a funeral, I at least want to wear the color-coordinated shoelaces I paid for.

When I got home from the hospital, I looked in textbooks to learn how to tie my laces one-handed. The instructions and drawings were hard to follow. Here is my attempt to do better. My detailed instructions make this task sound cumbersome, but I can tie my shoes so quickly now that therapists who have seen me do it have uttered an involuntary "wow."

Begin by re-lacing your shoes. The bottom hole you start with *must* make the lace come out of the last hole that is on your hemiplegic side (e.g., if your right side is your hemiplegic side, the lace must come out of the last hole on the right). When you thread the lace through the bottom hole, start at the center and go in the hole from the underside (see the arrow in Figure 1 on the next page). This hides the fuzzy little "pom-pom" that will form after you finish lacing your shoe and trim off the excess lace at the bottom. When you pull the lace through the bottom hole, leave a six to eight inch tail hanging out of the hole. You will need this tail so you can make the knot that anchors the lace. *Do not* knot the lace at the bottom *until* you tie your shoe one time to see if adjustments are needed. When you get to the top hole, leave six to eight inches of lace hanging out of the hole. You need enough lace at the top to tie the shoe plus some extra so you won't pull the lace out when you pull out the tongue to get your foot in the shoe.

If you use the same style of shoe year round as I do (tan in summer; black in winter), the re-lacing step can be streamlined once you figure out where to put the knots. I take the laces out of my old shoes, lay them next to the new laces, and use a pen to mark where to put the knots.

Figure 1.

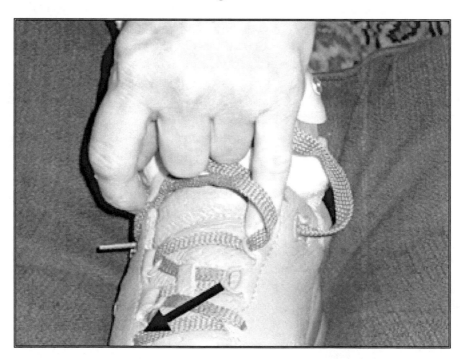

Tying Shoes One-Handed

Step 1. Pulling the lace tight.

Skip (1a) below *if* your shoe *only* has thick laces threaded through small holes punched in your shoe. When you pull thick laces through small holes, it creates friction that holds the laces tight after you let go so you won't need step 1a.

(1a) The lace coming out of the last grommet or D-ring needs to be pulled taut. Figure 1 shows you how to put tension on the lace by pressing down with the fingertip or knuckle of your ring or little finger. While pressing down on the lace with your ring or little finger, use your thumb and index finger to pull the slack through the hole on the opposite side. In Figure 1, you can see a sliver of my thumb behind my index finger getting ready to pull the lace taut.

(1b) Leave the lace that crosses horizontally between the top two holes loose so you can get your index finger under it in step 2.

Step 2. Making the 1ˢᵗ loop.

(2a) Grab the end of the lace with your last three fingers and slip your index finger under the top horizontal lace (see Figure 2 below). Your index finger should point towards your body. Use your index finger to snag the lace and drag it under the horizontal lace to make a messy looking loop.

Figure 2.

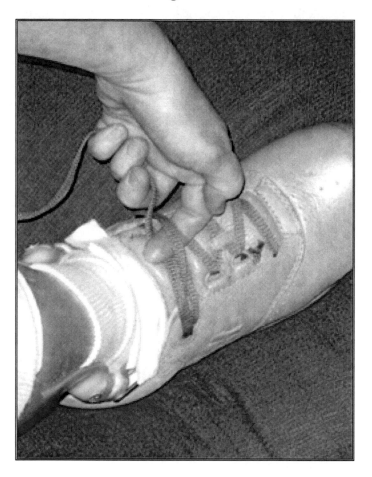

(2b) The top horizontal lace will be loose because your index finger was under it. An arrow in Figure 3 points at the hole where you need to pull the lace taut. Finish by pulling the messy looking lace into a neat looking loop.

Figure 3.

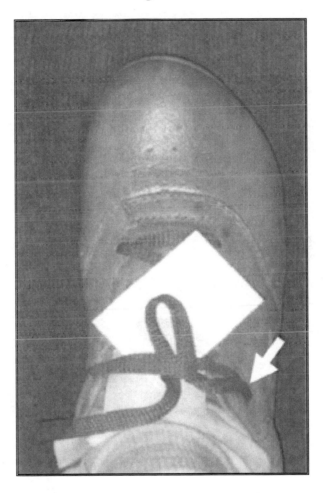

Step 3. Making a slipknot.

(3a) Grab the end of the lace with your fingers and use your thumb to push the lace through the 1st loop identified by the arrow in Figure 4. As you push your thumb through this loop, a 2nd loop will appear.

(3b) Pull your thumb out of the 1st loop. Grab the 2nd loop and yank it from side to side to tighten the slipknot you've just made.

Figure 4.

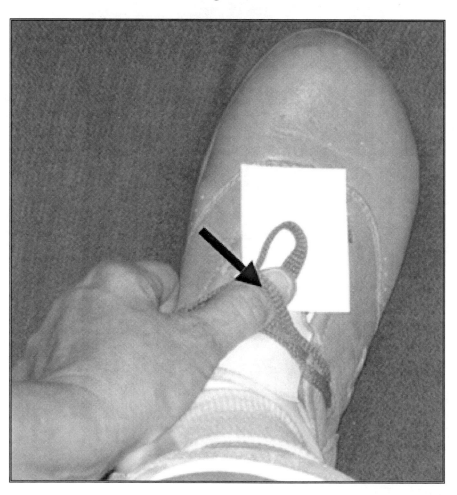

Step 4. Prevent tripping on the lace.

<u>For safety</u> use the excess lace to create a fake two-eared bow by threading the tip of the lace under the top horizontal lace *or* work the excess lace down to the bottom hole before you tie the knot that anchors the lace.

Now you are ready to tie a double knot at the bottom hole that anchors the lace. A Boy Scout leader told me this is a sailing knot that holds against great pressure. To tie a double knot, make two knots that lay *on top of* each other. If you make two knots that lay *side by side* like pearls on a necklace, the knot is more likely to come loose. Pull the knot tight. Cut off any excess lace at the bottom.

If you are not able or not interested in tying laces one-handed, you can buy jogging shoes with **Velcro** fastenings or an OT can make a Velcro closure for your shoes. Whatever shoes you decide to wear, you don't want to disrupt your grandchild's wedding by falling down and being taken away in an ambulance because your shoes were stylish but not securely fastened. To **prevent a fall**, consult with an OT before you make any changes in the way you fasten your shoes.

Don't Forget Outerwear

Not being able to fasten a coat really upsets me. No self-care task makes me feel more like a pre-schooler than picturing a friend and me standing in a restaurant while she zips up my coat. I wanted to learn how to zip my coat because I hate to be kept inside. As a child, I was a tomboy who ran outside to play as soon as I got home from school. My mother didn't have to nag me to do my homework after dinner. All she had to do was threaten to keep me in the house after school the next day. Growing up in Chicago also gave me the confidence to deal with bad weather. I walked a mile and a half to high school when it was forty degrees below freezing on the thermometer (not wind chill) while wearing a skirt and knee socks. This was back when girls weren't allowed to wear pants to school.

Three strategies make it easier to put on a coat. *First*, buy a short coat that has very little fabric below the zipper that you will have to hold out of the way. With a short coat, the hemiplegic hand doesn't need as much strength to hold the bottom edge of the coat as you join the zipper. Also look for coats that have a fabric tab that is attached to the end of the zipper tab. It's easier to grab a soft fabric tab than to grab a slippery metal tab. *Second*, double-check every step before you move on. Pull up on the first sleeve two or three times to make sure it is completely pulled up onto your hemiplegic shoulder as far as it will go. Then go back and make sure your hemiplegic hand is completely pulled through the sleeve opening. Only then should you reach behind you to put your sound arm in the second sleeve. Double-checking may be irritating at first, but it increases your chance of success on the first try. *Third*, donning a coat is easier if you use an adapted zipping procedure. This procedure has more steps than able-bodied people use, but I can't be in a bad mood when I'm outside.

Zipping a Coat in Three Steps

1. Getting Lined Up. Place the index finger of your sound hand along the bottom of the *joined* zipper. This index finger has to rest parallel to the bottom of the zipper and press up to keep the two ends of the zipper perfectly joined so the teeth won't get out of alignment. With your index finger pressing up, pinch the bottom of the coat between your sound thumb and middle finger to keep the coat still during Step 2.
2. Starting the Zipper. Grab the tab with your hemiplegic thumb and index finger and pull it up one inch to get the zipper started. Grabbing the tab is a struggle at the beginning of the winter, so I may (a) place rubber fingertips used to count money (available at Staples) on the thumb and index finger of my hemiplegic hand, (b) rehearse pinching without the zipper tab in my hand, or (c) press the back of my hand against something so my wrist bends and opens my hand.
3. Getting to the Top. After your hemiplegic hand gets the zipper started, reverse hand positions. Move your hemiplegic hand down to hold the bottom of the coat still while your sound hand finishes zipping all the way to the top.

You may wonder why I didn't ask my OT to put **Velcro** fastenings on my coats. The Velcro fastenings that came with my raincoat taught me their shortcomings. When you lean over to get in the car, pick up a package, or open a door, the coat gapes open between the squares of Velcro. When temperatures are in the 40s and 50s, losing a little body heat isn't that critical. However, when the temperature drops below freezing and the wind is blowing, I need a tightly closed coat. I suppose you could use long strips of Velcro, but I don't want to think about trying to line up a couple of feet of Velcro. I don't want my coat to look like it has been fastened by a young child.

New Jersey is sunny ten months of the year, so outerwear here includes sunglasses. It's difficult to don clip-on sunglasses one-handed. I use sunglasses that fit over my regular glasses, like the kind people wear after cataract surgery. You can quickly don these sunglasses after you come out of a tunnel or when it suddenly stops raining. I found a smaller pair at www.hammacher.com that matches the size of my prescription glasses. They are expensive but so quick and easy to put on and take off that they are worth it. I saw a cheaper pair at HDwraparound.com, but haven't tried them. I lost the first pair because I was always taking them off and putting them down. I have a thing about talking to people who can't see my eyes through dark sunglasses. I put the second pair on a strap that hangs around my neck. The neck strap made me feel old at first, but it gives me one less thing to manage when I go out, which helps me relax.

Finally, outerwear includes **winter boots**. You can't always avoid snow that is higher than the top of your street shoes. It may only take a trip from your front door to the car to leave you with wet, cold feet. If being homebound in the winter gives you cabin fever, there is hope. Here are some examples of what works and what doesn't.

A shoe salesman tried to shove my shoe into several boots with wide toes without success. A rigid brace can't straighten like an ankle does when you point your toes to slip your foot into a boot. So I bought two different types of plastic boots that fit over street shoes. Even getting them a size too big and slitting the plastic with a pair of scissors didn't give me enough slack to get my shoe with the brace inside the boot. My brace was too wide at the toe and too high at the arch.

Then I found a lightweight "overshoe" at plowandhearth.com that is worn over street shoes. This overshoe has a nylon upper with a long **Velcro** opening that goes all the way to the toe of the shoe. This long opening lets you maneuver a shoe with a rigid leg brace into the boot. After closing the front Velcro opening, the nylon fabric that protects the ankle is very full. To gather the excess fabric, you tighten a Velcro strap that goes around your ankle. This Velcro strap can be left long to accommodate the high arch of the brace. These Velcro fastenings allow the overshoe to fit snugly so you are not stumbling around in gigantic ill-fitting boots. These boots have good traction thanks to a thick rubber tread. The ankle-high version costs fifty dollars, but boots that keep your feet dry and don't take half an hour to put on are priceless.

You may not be as touchy as I am about having people put my coat on in public, but you will have to deal with outerwear sooner than you think. Doctors force you to leave your home by giving you prescriptions that are good for only thirty days after you leave rehab. My first visit to the doctor's office was in May, but the bad weather showed up eventually. Think of ways you can deal with outerwear.

Houdini Puts on a Bra One-Handed

It's odd to leave putting on a bra until the end of this chapter, but only desperate women will want to read this. If I were still married, I would probably have never figured out how to do this task. I am too large-breasted to slip a hooked bra over my head. Even an aide using her two good hands couldn't get a hooked bra past my large breasts. And don't talk to me about not wearing a bra. Clothes look terrible when your breasts are closer to your waist than you ever thought possible. When large breasts retire, they go south to Florida and come back up north to visit only when you wear a bra. Small-breasted women have the last laugh.

I worked very hard to learn how to put on a bra because I couldn't get past the idea of asking a friend to hook it. I couldn't imagine myself saying "I'd love to come for dinner if you would hook my bra when I get there." This problem is not discussed in the one-handed literature, so I hope this information helps other large-breasted women. My method involves using a clothespin to hook your bra in front, turning the bra around, and pulling it up.

This adapted procedure begins by preparing the bra. In summer, cornstarch makes it easier to slide the bra around. I like cornstarch because it is odorless. A shaker designed for confectioner's sugar is a good container for any fine-grained product. Rubbing cornstarch on your body one-handed is messy, but rubbing it on the bra isn't. To make sure that only a small amount comes flying out, fill the container half full, lay the container on its side, and gently tap the container on the bra instead of shaking it. Then rub the cornstarch into the bra. In winter, I have the opposite problem. When my skin is dry, the shoulder straps repeatedly fall off my shoulders. I solve this problem by putting my bra on, slipping the shoulder straps down, and squirting a dab of hand lotion from a pump dispenser where the straps rest.

To fasten the bra while sitting, clip a clothespin on to the eyelet end of the bra. Stick the handles of the clothespin under the elastic waistband of your underpants on the hemiplegic side of your navel. Putting the clothespin slightly off center puts your hand in the midline. This makes it easier to see what you are doing. If the clothespin twists the bra fabric, smooth it flat. Now you are ready to flip the hook end of the bra behind you. When you pull the hook end around to the front, the clothespin and friction from your skin are enough to hold the bra still while you fasten the first hook. Good lighting is essential for hooking the bra. Just raking the hook across the eyelet doesn't work. Start by grasping the hook end between your thumb and index finger. To put a hook through its eyelet, grasp the hook with your thumb and index finger and slip your middle finger under the eyelet section. When the hook is directly over the eyelet, press down on the hook and push up on the eyelet section as you slide the two together. Once the top hook is fastened, remove the clothespin and hook the rest of the eyelets.

To finish, turn the bra around so the hooks are in back. I unhooked my bra as I was turning it around the first few times and almost gave up. When turning the bra around, be sure to grab the fabric as far away as you can from the hooks you just fastened. Then put your arms under the straps (hemiplegic arm first) and slip them halfway up your arms. To get the bra all the way up, lay your sound forearm horizontally underneath both cups, push the bra up, and pull the shoulder straps up the rest of the way. If the shoulder straps are twisted and <u>it is safe for you</u>, lean forward in sitting with your hemiplegic arm dangling between your legs to take weight off the straps. You can also slip a finger under the straps where they attach in back to untwist them.

After months of practice, I can execute this procedure quickly and effortlessly. It took me longer to master this self-care task than any other, but wearing a bra in public is worth it to me. I've even learned to don it when I'm out. After asking a nurse to hook my sweaty bra after a doctor's physical exam, I learned to keep a clothespin in my purse. The clothespin comes in handy when dressing after an x-ray, a mammogram, etc. If you need to put on a bra one-handed, it is possible.

The Bottom Line

I didn't write this long chapter to give you a long to-do list. I hope you gave yourself permission to skip the sections you were not interested in. Stroke survivors ultimately decide which self-care tasks they will do when they go home. But don't shoot yourself in the foot. If the people who are helping you become exhausted, you are shaving months or even years off of the time they can keep you at home. When family members believe they have to do everything for a loved one who has had a stroke, they often get so worn out that they become sick. That's when doctors start talking about putting one person in the hospital and the other person in a nursing home.

Think outside the box. If I get tired in the middle of the day, I leave my shoes and leg brace on and lie down on top of my bedspread. This allows me to get up without having to put my shoes and brace back on. My mother taught me not to put my shoes on the bed, but who am I saving that twenty-year-old bedspread for? When I find a new bedspread I like, I'll spread an old towel over the end of the bed where my shoes are. When you enter an institution, you have to follow everyone else's rules. Don't waste the freedom that living at home gives you by getting stuck on the fact that you can't do self-care the way you've always done it.

CHAPTER 5

ADVANCED ADLs IN THE HOME

Advanced Activities of Daily Living (ADLs) are more than cleaning the house. They include paying bills, changing burnt out light bulbs, and taking your medications properly. I was astounded by the number of advanced ADL tasks that had to be taken care of even before I got home. When you are admitted to the hospital, family and friends want to call you. Honey, the hospital doesn't turn on the phone until they see the money. That means someone has to hightail it to the business office or give you cash so you are ready when the phone lady shows up.

My friends divided up the advanced ADLs I needed help with while I was still in the hospital. Bobbie drove past the rehab hospital on her way to work, so she **volunteered** to do my laundry every week and bring me cash. Greg made a detour on the way home from work to pick up the mail at my house and give the bills to Arlene, who lives two blocks from him. I didn't have to worry about an overdue mortgage payment or late fees on my credit cards because Arlene volunteered to write checks while I was in the hospital. She forged my signature and every company took my money without any questions. Amazingly, no one cared that my signature suddenly looked different as long as they got my money.

Then a terrible experience in the hospital gave me the courage I needed to take care of my home. The staff trusted me to wheel myself to and from therapy, but one day I made the mistake of wheeling my chair outside to sit with other patients after my last treatment. An aide eventually found me and said I couldn't sit outside without a family member to supervise me. When I pointed out that other patients didn't have family members with them, she spun my wheelchair around and firmly propelled me back to the nursing floor. I was outraged. I was probably three years old the last time my mother dragged me by the hand to bring me back inside. I held my tongue and went to the psychologist who negotiated a deal with the nursing staff. I had to come back to the nursing floor and sign out when I wanted to go anywhere besides therapy. This mortifying experience turned out to be a blessing in disguise. When I worried about going home to live alone, I would think about this incident and get angry instead.

A Small Army Got Me into My New Home

My story took an unusual turn because I had to sell my house while I was still in the rehabilitation hospital. My old house had one bathroom on the second floor and I couldn't repeatedly climb the steep steps. I had been meaning to sell the house for five years, but the housing market was depressed. I had been advised by several realtors to expect a loss of at least $20,000. A friend recommended a realtor who came to the hospital. Then a miracle happened. My house sold on the first day, sight unseen, for more than my asking price. In the meantime, my friend Peggy went on the Internet, found a gorgeous new trailer with cathedral ceilings, central air, and a full-size laundry room. I signed out of the rehab hospital and Peggy and her husband John took me to see it.

Of course, real estate deals don't close when you want them to, so I had to sell my old house before my new house was ready. I put all my belongings in storage and my friend Arlene put me in her spare bedroom for what turned out to be three months. We split the expenses, but Arlene did the grocery shopping, cooked dinner, and had a housekeeper do the cleaning.

It took more **volunteers** to get me into my new home. My brothers Mark and Jim volunteered to fly out from Illinois to pack up my old house. My friends Ann and Joanne volunteered to drive from Wisconsin to unpack my new house. Anne loves to decorate, so she volunteered to help me pick out carpeting, wallpaper, and countertops. Peggy, who also loves to decorate, volunteered to take me shopping, helped me choose drapes, and hung them. Suzanne volunteered to drive me to places I needed to be until I qualified for Paratransit services for the handicapped. John, a computer programmer, volunteered to set up my computer in my new home and fixed computer glitches. Bobbie and Greg volunteered to take me grocery shopping to stock my new kitchen and carried two shopping carts' worth of stuff into my house.

Baby Steps Come First

When my friends closed the front door and left me alone, I was only marginally terrified because I had taken baby steps while I was living with my friend Arlene. She helped me by giving me honest feedback instead of hiding my mistakes from me. She made me aware of my errors in a matter-of-fact tone that made it easy to accept her feedback. Here is one example. The first time I used her shower, I got water all over the rug. Instead of sneaking the rug downstairs to dry and then sneaking it back up to the bathroom, she told me what I had done. She said I would do better next time and because of her feedback I did. Making a mess that I would have to clean up when I lived alone suddenly came up on my radar. Most people would have tried to do everything for me, but Arlene helped me think about homecare early.

After awareness came skill. Arlene helped me get downstairs in the morning and then had to open her shop so I made myself a peanut butter sandwich for breakfast and a meat sandwich for lunch. Fortunately, while I was in rehab my OT had made sure I could get food out of the refrigerator, open a can of soda, and make a sandwich. Arlene liked to have a clean kitchen table when she cooked dinner. I made sure my numerous papers, like medical bills, were put away every night. I washed the mug I used every day. I put my empty soda can in the recycling bin. These are small tasks that a child can do, but they were symbolic of my determination to be independent. Succeeding safely at these simple tasks gave me confidence that I could take care of myself in my own home.

An old life lesson also helped me be less afraid of tackling homecare. In the hospital, I worried for four weeks about how I was going to get ice cubes out of a tray one-handed. Then I remembered having told my students that making a movie in your head is the hardest way to solve a concrete problem. It's easier to solve the problem when you have the equipment. Once I had the ice cube tray in my hand, I discovered the solution. After an ice cube tray reminded me that objects teach us how to manipulate them, I stopped obsessing about how I was going to take care of my home.

Mom, Answer the Phone

My telephone skills were jump-started by selling my old house, buying a new home, and making arrangements to be moved. However, every stroke survivor who has to be left alone for a little while needs to master this task. When a caregiver runs errands, everyone wants to know you can use the telephone.

You begin by getting to the phone. Putting a telephone in every room can **prevent a fall** because you won't have to race to answer a phone in the next room. I have a phone close to my bed, my dining room table, and my computer. Can't get up from the couch fast enough? Don't worry – caller ID lets you call the person right back. Scroll down the list of missed calls until you get to the most recent one and hit the make-a-call button. The phone will dial the number for you. If you buy a cordless phone and <u>can walk safely and independently</u> with a cane or walker, you may be able to **transport** the phone to a more convenient location. Place the phone in a small bag tied on your walker. If you walk with a cane, put the phone in your hemiplegic armpit or hand or put it in a small bag that is Velcroed to your cane (see the next section on transporting objects). Carry the phone to the couch to have long talks with friends and family. Carry it to the kitchen table where you can sit to take a message. If transporting the phone is unrealistic, make sure you have a place to sit down or furniture arrangements that are **wheelchair accessible**.

Taking messages was a challenge at first. Repeatedly putting down the phone receiver so I could write down information was frustrating. Using my sound shoulder to press the receiver up to my ear while I wrote didn't work either. I had to ask people to repeat themselves because my shoulder couldn't keep the receiver tight against my ear. Just writing down a phone number was a trial for both me and the person on the other end of the line.

I didn't want to use a speakerphone. The few times I've used one, I felt silly talking to a box. I wanted a headset that went over the top of my head, but a friend talked me into buying an ear bud that fits over my ear lobe. I wasn't wild about the idea, but I went along with her. The ear bud is easy to put on one-handed, comfortable to wear, and doesn't mess up my hair. I was sold. Somebody is going to have to pry it off my cold dead body. Even better, leave the ear bud on when you put me in the casket so my family and friends can call me until my cell phone battery goes dead.

With the ear bud on, you can write down phone messages with your sound hand. To keep the paper from slipping, put a piece of clear **Dycem** under the paper. Clear Dycem is smooth. It was designed specifically for writing. You can order it at www.sammonspreston.com. Clear Dycem works better than a clipboard that doesn't always stay still and is cantankerous when you try to slip the paper under the clip. I have a piece of clear Dycem and a pen next to every telephone in my house. A ballpoint pen isn't very forgiving because you have to hold the pen at just the right angle to make the ink flow. I recommend gel pens like the Pilot G-2, which I buy in bulk at Staples. They are more expensive than ballpoint pens, but they last a long time.

The telephone solutions you come up with to meet your particular needs may be different from mine. Whatever you do, don't skimp on your telephone setup. The telephone is your lifeline, but it doesn't do you any good if you can't use it.

Taking Meds Wrong Can Kill You

For safety, skip this section on taking medication if you don't have the vision and cognitive ability to use the memory aids described below. I've taken lots of vitamins for years, but that didn't prepare me for keeping track of all the pills I have to take since my stroke. I thought I knew my medications because I had been taking them in the hospital for two months, but the nurses were doing the thinking. When I took over the job at home, it was confusing because several pills look similar. There is the orange oval pill, the pink oval pill, the pink round pill, etc. Taking my medications correctly can prevent another stroke so I take the following procedures very seriously.

The only way to deal with medications is to be organized. I began by creating a cheat sheet that lists the color and shape of every pill as well as drug names, dosages, and times I take them. I had to look at this **memory aid** for several weeks. Another memory aid is keeping your prescription bottles in a cheap food container. You don't have to worry about taking the wrong bottles out of the medicine cabinet because they are together in their own container. I keep the food container in a kitchen cabinet so I can sit at the kitchen table to transfer pills from the pharmacy bottles to a seven-day container. Using a pillbox with seven compartments is another memory aid. The compartments are labeled with the days of the week so you know what pills to take each day. Using this container means you rack your brains and open all those bottles once a week instead of every day. I was eventually able to fill this weekly pillbox without looking at my cheat sheet. Pill recognition is such a relief.

When you go out, you won't want to lug a big purse around that holds a big pillbox with all your pills for the week. Each morning, I transfer one day's supply of pills to a small pillbox. Make the transfer one-handed by placing the one-day pillbox upside down on top of the compartment for that day. Hold the two containers firmly together and quickly flip them so the one-day container is now on the bottom. A few pills may spill on the countertop, but with practice you will get good at this. To get pills out of the one-day pillbox, put it on a piece of **non-slip shelf liner**. The pillbox will stay still when you reach in to get a pill. You may prefer to use a different set of pill containers. Visit a drugstore to find pill containers that are suited to your needs.

Grouping is another **memory aid** that will help you take your medications correctly. When taking several pills at one time, assume you will make mistakes. One way to check is to create small groups of pills after you take them out of the pillbox. For example, in the morning I take three blood pressure pills, two cholesterol pills, and two pills for miscellaneous conditions (hyperthyroidism; allergies). People use this grouping strategy when they group cards they've been dealt into suits. While I put the suits of cards in any order in my hand, I always put my groups of pills in the same order on the table. I create a straight line by putting cholesterol pills on the left, blood pressure pills on the right, and miscellaneous pills in the middle. Think of a way to group your pills that makes sense to you and triggers your memory. *Always* check to make sure you have taken out the correct pills before you swallow them.

Location is another **memory aid**. After you take your morning meds, put your pillbox in a location that will help you remember to take them. If I am going out, I lay the one-day pillbox next to my driving glasses to remind me to put the pillbox in my purse. On the days I stay home, I put the pillbox on the cart I use to **transport** my meals to the table. Think about locations that will help you take your medicine on time.

My final memory aid is to print out a list of my drugs that I give other people. This list includes the names, dosages, and number of times I take a pill each day. My primary physician told me it is distressing to get a call from the emergency room at two in the morning when no one knows what kind or how much medication her patient has taken that day. Always carry a couple of copies of your drug list in your wallet or purse to give away. Everybody wants them. Every time you see a doctor, nurse, or therapist, they want to know what medications you are taking. Health-care providers are happy to get a typed list because they don't have to rely on my memory. I am happy because I don't have to keep writing out this darn list over and over. If you can't type up a drug list, have someone do it for you and have them print out several copies.

Transporting Objects without Taking All Day

Wherever you are, the things you need always seem to be in the place you just came from. This is a constant source of irritation because you may have to make multiple trips, carrying one object at a time. Argh! The alternative is to use bags and carts. The solutions are relatively inexpensive. Look up transporting objects in the Index to see how often this problem comes up.

A cane monopolizes the only trustworthy hand a stroke survivor has, so **transporting** objects while walking with a cane can be a challenge. To carry light objects from room to room, put them in a small bag. I began with small gift bags from the card section, but these paper bags didn't hold up. Now I use a 7 x 9½-inch nylon tote bag that I found at Barnes & Noble. Stick self-adhesive **Velcro** on your cane and on the bag so the bag won't bang against your cane as you walk.

This small bag allows you to carry the remote control, a wireless telephone, and many other small objects.

It's safer to transport a large object or several small objects with a **rolling cart**. A cart with horizontal wire baskets keeps objects from rolling off the cart as you push it from room to room. This cart rolls easily over carpeting. It can be purchased at www.organizeit.com or www.walmart.com. I use it to straighten a room by gathering all the clutter I need to put away.

To transport objects in the kitchen, you need a rolling cart that has solid shelves. When I was able-bodied I made many trips to the refrigerator to get items one at a time. This is too tiring after a stroke. A cart trails behind me while I load up food from the refrigerator to take to the countertop. It carries dirty dishes from the table to the sink. It transports hot dishes safely if you keep a large heat-resistant mat on the top shelf. Fatigue has taught me to check the area I'm in and make sure my cart is loaded up before I move on.

Bill Collectors Don't Care If You Have a Stroke

This section describes bill paying, but you may be able to use the procedures below to open personal mail, like letters and cards. I knew that paying bills requires good cognitive skills but never thought about the manual dexterity it also requires.

Learning to open an envelope took trial and error. Using a one-handed suction-cup letter opener didn't work. Dragging an envelope through the device broke the suction every time. When I stood and trapped an envelope by pressing down on the table with my whole hemiplegic hand, the letter opener dragged the envelope out from under my hand. I didn't become proficient at opening envelopes until I made an accidental discovery. One day I was opening my mail at the kitchen table and plunked an envelope down on the rubber placemat I use to keep my plate still while eating. Without thinking, I folded the placemat over the top of the envelope. Now the edge of the envelope was the "meat" in a rubber placemat sandwich. At your desk, fold a piece of **non-slip shelf liner** around the envelope before you press down to hold it still.

I used my teeth to get bills and letters out of their envelopes for quite a while, but who knows where my mail has been. My post office was the one that was contaminated by anthrax. Authorities have cleaned up the anthrax, but what else is being transferred from one envelope to the next by the sorting machines? I regained the ability to hold an envelope between my hemiplegic thumb and fingers, but don't have enough strength to hold an envelope still when I pull out a multi-page bill or a tight fitting card. If you have a similar problem, try folding a small piece of non-slip shelf liner over the edge of the envelope to increase friction. If you can stand safely without holding on to something, try standing to get mail out of envelopes. You don't have to lift your arm as high to hold the envelope in standing as you do when you sitting.

Dycem and a stapler can help you handle checks and pay stubs. Put a generous square of clear **Dycem** on the desk or table where you pay your bills to provide friction as you write. To keep a ledger open when you enter checks, place a stapler on the upper edge of the opened ledger and your hemiplegic hand on the lower edge. To tear a pay stub off of a bill, pre-crease the fold line and place a stapler next to the tear line. Even a stapler isn't heavy enough to hold the paper still when you tear so press down on the stapler with your whole hand. For safety, position your fingers over the *back* end of the stapler where the hinge is so your fingers won't get caught in the stapler when it closes. Using a stapler to tear a dotted line beats taping a ripped pay stub back together. To get the pay stub and check in the envelope one-handed, place the envelope on **Dycem**, which holds the envelope still as you wiggle the check and pay stub side-to-side to slide them in. To draw a line in your checkbook to show where the last statement period ended, run a pencil along the edge of the stapler instead of a ruler.

In addition to Dycem and a stapler, adapted procedures can help you handle checks and pay stubs as well. The *first* procedure is the **backwards rule**, which is described in Chapter Four on self-care. While practicing on mock checks I got from my recreational therapist while I was in the hospital, I discovered that making the letter "c" from the bottom up made it more legible than making it from the top down. Starting on the line and moving the pen upwards guarantees that letters won't go below the line. If you have to learn how to print with your non-dominant hand, see if drawing some letters backwards ensures your early success. Printing legibly with a non-dominant hand takes patience, but being able to write checks and sign credit card slips is important because a girl's got to shop.

The **backwards rule** can help you handle paperwork, like stapling the multiple pages that come with some bills. One hand can bring the stapler to paper, but the stapler can knock some sheets out of alignment if your other hand doesn't hold the stack together. Then the stapler may not catch every sheet. Instead, use the backwards rule to staple. Position the stapler and bring the stack of papers to the stapler. Filing a bill in a folder one-handed is easier if you hold the bill by the edge of the paper that goes in first. Push your whole hand in the folder to keep it open so you can see what you are doing.

A *second* procedure that makes bill paying easier is using an assembly line process. Before my stroke, I used to go through all the steps with one bill and then repeat the process with each subsequent bill. When I was able-bodied, I wasn't aware that shuffling all this paper around requires a lot of fine-motor skill. Now I complete one step for every bill in the stack, like writing all the checks before stuffing all the return envelopes.

These solutions address only the fine-motor components of paying bills. You have to decide if you have the cognitive skills to resume this task. The consequences of making errors while paying bills are expensive. Late fees are big and bill collectors are not going to forgive mistakes because you had a stroke.

A Computer isn't a Luxury

I wanted to learn how to use the computer one-handed because I use it for so many things. I use it to print a current list of my medications, send e-mails, write letters to insurance companies, track my monthly finances, keep an updated list of addresses for Paratransit, and a host of other tasks. Writing this book would have been impossible without a computer. I can print legibly, but it's slow and makes my hand cramp up.

The first typing skill I had to relearn was to hit the space bar between words. I kept forgetting this simple step because I was focusing so intensely on finding the letters. Learning to touch type in high school helped me memorize where every key is without looking, but this knowledge was useless when I was forced to type one-handed. Saying each letter silently as I typed helped because it slowed me down when I was looking for the correct keys. Another useful skill is knowing easy ways to move the cursor around. The mouse can move the cursor to a specific spot on the page, but letting go of the mouse at just the right instant is tricky. It is faster and more accurate to move the cursor around by using the arrow keys to get to the place you want to be. You can also move the cursor quickly to the left margin by pressing the Home key and move it quickly to the right margin by pressing the End key.

A member of my stroke support group said his friends on the Internet complained that he was shouting because he typed everything with the Caps Lock key on. I have a small hand, but I can simultaneously press two keys to type capital letters one-handed. Those piano lessons I took as a child turned out to be useful. There is a Shift key on either side of the keyboard. I use my little finger or index finger to hold down the closest Shift key while another finger presses a letter key to make a capital letter. If this is too difficult, you can activate a software program called Sticky Keys, which is installed at the factory on many computers. This program recognizes when you want one key held down while you press a second key at the same time. To access Sticky Keys, click on Control Panel and look for the Accessibility option. It took hours of practice, but I can type faster than some able-bodied people who peck at the keyboard with two index fingers.

If you spend a lot of time at your computer, using equipment that ensures **good positioning** cuts down on back and neck pain. Office supply stores sell adjustable chairs. Look for the following features. On a good chair, the seat goes up and down to adjust the height of the seat from the floor. This allows you to keep your flat feet on the floor and the monitor at eye level so you don't crane your neck by looking up. You should be able to adjust the tilt of the backrest so your back is erect. The armrest height should be adjustable so your hemiplegic elbow is supported. I always position my hand when I work at the computer by resting it on the platform that holds my keyboard. I also have computer glasses. The entire lens has one prescription for the eighteen-inch distance to the monitor. I don't have to crane my neck to look through the middle section of tri-focals or constantly turn my head side-to-side to scan to the edges of the monitor.

Since my computer was set up for a right-handed person, everything had to be switched so I could use my sound left hand. The world doesn't cater to left-handed people, so you will have to be creative if you have a similar problem. Here is one way to do it. I already had a pullout keyboard shelf that is attached to my computer desk. This shelf adjusts the height and tilt of the keyboard. A friend, Joanne, unscrewed this pull-out shelf and reattached it on the left side of my computer desk. This pullout keyboard now sits next to a narrow table on my left side where my mouse and mouse pad are placed. This eighteen-inch wide table is designed to fit behind a couch. The shelf is big enough to hold my keyboard and support my hemiplegic right hand while my hemiplegic arm rests at my side.

Using a computer after a stroke requires multiple solutions. Buying good positioning equipment and computer glasses is some of the best money I've ever spent. For me, having a computer is a necessity rather than a luxury. Of course, if you don't use the computer as much as I do, you will want to spend your money on something else.

I'm Not Washing My Clothes at a Laundromat

Doing the laundry is a challenge because it never ends and can't be put off when you are out of clean clothes. A family member can't always run over to your house on the day you run out of clean clothes, so think about how to deal with this task. A feature that made me choose a trailer is that I have a laundry room on the first floor. Going down to the basement or walking to another building in bad weather is unthinkable for me. Even carrying a loaded laundry basket to another room is <u>not safe for me</u>. If you don't have to carry clothes up and down stairs and can afford some equipment, you may be able to do the laundry.

A **rolling cart** with three wire baskets lets you put different colored clothes in different baskets and transport the dirty clothes to the laundry room. The cart is available at www.organizeit.com or www.Walmart.com. For safety, keep a chair close to the dirty clothes hamper so you can sit as you sort the dirty clothes and load them on the cart. If you need a **cane** or **walker** to keep from leaning on the cart for support, you can push the cart a foot or so ahead of you and walk up to it.

For safety, keep another chair in the laundry room so you can sit down as you pull clothes out of the dryer. It may be unsafe for you to lean forward in sitting to reach for clothes in the *back* of the dryer. If leaning this far forward puts you **at risk for falling**, use a long-handled reacher to pull the clothes to the front of the dryer where you can pull them out by hand while sitting erect. While sitting in front of the dryer, load the dry clothes on the top basket of your cart so it is ready to roll back to the bedroom.

Folding clothes on the bed is easy. You have plenty of room to lay the clothes flat, fold them over, and stack the folded clothes as you go along. To hang shirts on a hanger, stick your whole hemiplegic hand into one sleeve to hold the shirt in the air and then slip the hanger in the neck and one sleeve. You have to hold the shirt that is halfway on the hanger so your sound hand can slide the hanger in the other sleeve. Hold on to the shirt by pinching the shoulder area with your hemiplegic fingers or using your whole hand to press the garment against your stomach. Fold pants over your hemiplegic forearm and slip the bottom of the pant legs onto the hanger.

When I first moved into my home, I tried to fold sheets. The only way I could fold a queen-size sheet was to open it completely and lay it lengthwise on the bed. Then I had to fold it in half again and again. This took so many trips around the bed that I finally gave up. Now I wad a matching top and bottom sheet into a bundle and put it on a shelf. My clean sheets are wrinkled, but the pressure of fitting them over my mattress smoothes them out enough to make me happy. I still fold pillowcases and my company's bed linen. No one is going to put me in a nursing home because my sheets are wrinkled. You might consider compromising as I did.

A Microwave Oven Saves the Day

I considered Meals on Wheels, but there are several drawbacks to this service. They don't supply meals on the weekends, so I would have to prepare some food anyway. They provide the hot meal at lunch, which meant I would have to arrange my entire schedule to be home in the middle of the day if I wanted to eat the food while it was hot. A cold meal is provided in the evening, but I can make my own sandwiches. Meals on Wheels is a valuable respite service for family members who cook for a homebound stroke survivor on weekdays, but it didn't meet my needs.

When I moved into my new home, I microwaved frozen dinners for two months. If it is <u>not safe for you to handle hot objects, skip this section</u> on the microwave oven. You need good safety awareness and hot/cold discrimination when you cook food in a microwave oven.

Frozen dinners are expensive, repetitive (lots of chicken), and have a lot of salt. When frozen dinners became boring, my first goal was to cook real food using the microwave over my stove. This required me to handle glass dishware. I couldn't use large glass dishes because they are too heavy for me to lift one-handed. Even now that I can lift light objects with two hands, I don't trust my hemiplegic hand to hold a hot, heavy dish.

Surprisingly, I can't get small glass dishes in and out of the microwave oven either. The problem is that the lid on the glass dish slides off when I lift the covered dish with one hand. I wanted to put plastic wrap on my glass dishes, but plastic wrap is hard to handle even when you have two good hands.

I found a device that makes handling plastic wrap a breeze. The device, called the "food wrap box," is available at www.solutions.com. It is shaped like a regular box of plastic wrap, but is made of hard plastic and has serrated teeth that are sharper than a store-bought box. <u>For safety</u>, keep your hands off of the serrated cutting teeth. Place the food wrap box next to your glass dish and open the lid. Pull out some plastic wrap, keeping constant tension on the plastic to keep the food wrap box pulled tight against the dish. Close the food wrap box to cut the plastic wrap. No tearing by hand is required. The plastic wrap isn't quite centered on the dish, but it's easy to reposition because it is stretched out flat on the rim of the dish. Center the plastic, smooth the sides down to seal the dish, and slit a hole in the top to let steam escape. <u>For safety, put on hot mitts</u> when you remove the hot dish from the microwave. To drain the water, leave the plastic wrap in place, pick up the dish with hot mitts, and tilt the dish in the sink. Water leaks out from under the plastic wrap so you don't have to use a strainer. Carefully pull the plastic wrap back so the steam doesn't scald you.

Food Prep with Low and High Tech Solutions

I finally got bored enough with microwaved food to try some simple cooking, like making scrambled eggs, a hamburger, and pasta with spaghetti sauce from a jar. I was cooking one food at a time and eating it from the pot I had cooked it in. I'll never forget the night I got three foods ready at the same time and put them on a plate. This milestone took four months to achieve because I had to practice every one-handed technique many times before I could work fast enough to think about how to get an entire meal ready at once. On December 10th, I realized that if I did this step first and that step second, all the food would be ready at the same time. So I thought I might as well celebrate by putting them together on a plate. I only reheated sliced roast beef with canned mushroom gravy. It wasn't gourmet cooking, but with green beans and a baked potato, the food looked nice together. Aesthetics requires a brain that isn't bogged down with details. Whether you eat dishes one at a time or can serve an entire meal at once, homemade meals are less boring and cheaper than eating frozen dinners. And you don't have to lie to your doctor about eating healthy.

Gadgets for food prep that are Wal-Mart cheap. By accident, I discovered cheap low-tech kitchen gadgets that help with food preparation. When you flip food with a spatula or stir hot food one-handed, you end up pushing the pot off the burner. <u>For safety, place a hot pot on</u> a fabric hot plate or a hot mitt that is sitting on the counter. The roughness of the fabric and weight of the pot create enough friction to hold the pot still while you stir or flip. A fabric hot plate also allows you to slide hot dishes across the countertop. Cheap, flexible ice cube trays are the easiest to bend when you empty them. Cut up lettuce for a salad by placing one leaf at a time on a cutting board and rolling over each leaf with a pizza cutter. Once you remove the twist tie from a new loaf of bread, the pointed end of an old-fashioned hand-held can opener can help you rip open the inner plastic lining. The lid from a peanut butter jar makes measuring spices and cooking oil less messy. Place a measuring spoon in the upside-down lid. Resting the handle of a measuring spoon on the rim keeps the spoon relatively level and the lid catches any spills.

Expensive gadgets help you chop and cut. If it is <u>not safe for you to handle knives, skip this section </u>on chopping and cutting. Even a food processor requires you to chop food into big pieces by hand before you put them in the processor. You need good safety awareness to safely chop meat and vegetables.

I am on a low-salt, low-fat diet, so being able to cut up chicken and season food with garlic, onions and other vegetables is a life-and-death issue. That's why I love my Etac Deluxe One-Handed cutting board. This cutting board has a group of nine thin nails placed in a square configuration so you can impale meat when cutting it into pieces or trimming off fat. The nails are embedded in a small removable section of the cutting board you can put in the dishwasher to kill bacteria. I cut up a large skinless chicken breast by cutting it into fourths crosswise before I cut it into small strips lengthwise.

The part of the cutting board I use the most is the adjustable vise. The vise gently holds soft foods, like tomatoes, for slicing. Don't worry about coring tomatoes. It's easier to cut the core out of each individual slice. The vise can trap a slice of bread so you can spread food like mustard. The vise can be removed to wash off food.

The vise firmly holds harder foods, but it takes two hands to cut through them. <u>For safety, you must</u> use a large knife and be able to make a fist with your hemiplegic hand! This allows you to use the heel of your hemiplegic hand to push down near the tip of the big knife while keeping your fingers away from the blade. Using this adapted procedure allows me to safely cut hard food, like apples or onions. Suction cups hold the cutting board still as I cut hard food, but they have better suction when they are wet. After I cut a bagel halfway down, I loosen the vise slightly to make it easier to finish cutting to the bottom. The two parts of the vise can be pulled ten inches apart so it accommodates even large pieces of food, like an entire head of lettuce.

The Etac Deluxe cutting board (also called the Swedish cutting board) is more expensive than other cutting boards designed for one-handed people. Yet it has so many uses that I think the expense is worth it. A trip to the emergency room after cutting yourself is much more expensive. The Etac cutting board is available at www.sammmonspreston.com.

A food processor is great, but it took some experimenting to use one-handed. For safety, never grab a food processor blade near the cutting surface because it is extremely sharp. When you use the pulse feature, the blade cuts vegetables into uneven-size pieces from big chunks to minutely minced pieces. A food processor chops best when you use the slicing blade.

To chop celery, I start by using my Etac cutting board to help me manually cut the celery into short thin strips. Then I put the slicing blade in the machine and place the strips vertically in the small tube with the round opening. I stuff the opening from both sides until it is firmly packed so the pieces won't fall out as I tilt the tube into place. Slicing thin strips produces small uniform pieces. This works for chopping baby carrots too.

To chop a *small* quantity of onions, green peppers, or cucumbers for a single salad or sandwich, I manually cut the food into big chunks, put the slicing blade in the machine, and put pieces of food in the wider oval-shaped tube opening. I put the sliced vegetables into a storage container, take out the small quantity I need, and run over the slices with the pizza cutter to get smaller pieces.

Emptying a food processor requires some tricks. I have high countertops so I would have to hold the food processor container high in the air to empty it. It's easier to transfer food from the food processor to a storage container if I place the storage container on my **kitchen cart**, which is lower. After dumping out the contents, finish emptying the food processor by trapping the container between your stomach and your whole hemiplegic hand with the handle pushed against your waist *or* by grabbing the handle with your hemiplegic fingers and pressing the container against your stomach. Once you have a secure grasp on the container, use your sound hand to scoop out the food that sticks to the inside walls of the container.

To chop a *large* quantity of onions for a pot of spaghetti sauce or chili, I use another gadget called an Alligator Vegetable Chopper. It is available at Williams-Sonoma stores, but there are cheaper knock-offs at many discount stores. The Alligator has a sharp cutting grid, but you still have to push down quickly and forcefully to chop an onion. I lean on the Alligator with my hemiplegic elbow as I push down with my sound hand. This device works best if you cut a medium-sized onion in half pole to pole and then cut each half into four pieces so you are putting only one-eighth of an onion in the chopper a at a time. The two parts of the Alligator Vegetable Chopper come apart easily and are dishwasher safe. But be careful! The cutting grid will deceive you. If you grab the cutting grid at one angle, the blade feels dull while at another angle it is as sharp as the dickens. <u>For safety, keep your hands off the cutting grid at all times</u>. When food gets stuck in the cutting grid, I use eyebrow tweezers I keep in the kitchen that are dedicated to this task.

I've tried pre-chopped garlic in a jar and I think it's nasty. If you love garlic as much as I do, here is how you get fresh, chopped garlic. Loosen the skin from a clove by smashing it with the bottom of a small glass custard cup. Chop a garlic clove with a large chef's knife. The handle and the blade of a *paring* knife are in a straight line, but a *chef's* knife is bigger and the handle is an inch or two wider than the blade. This keeps your fingers from hitting the cutting board as you rock the knife up and down to cut a piece of food. Slice the clove lengthwise, lay the two halves flat, and then slice it into strips. Turn the strips 90 degrees so you can chop them crosswise. Then just keep going over the garlic until the pieces get progressively smaller. This takes time and a few pieces are bigger than I would like. Bigger pieces taste milder when cooked so I don't worry about it.

<u>It isn't safe for me</u> to pick up a pile of chopped food by pushing the food against the blade of a knife. I pick up chopped food by holding a dough scraper in my hemiplegic hand while my sound hand pushes the food up onto the dough scraper. Both hands transport the dough

scraper that is loaded up with food to a pot or storage container. This cheap kitchen device eliminates a lot of frustration. It can take quite a while to transfer chopped food by picking up a few pieces at a time with your sound hand. Little pieces of cut-up garlic are especially slippery. People could hear me shout in the next state when I discovered this trick.

Cleaning Varies from Easy to Difficult

Losing the freedom of living in my home because I can't clean it is a severe consequence. Many health-care agencies don't provide homecare assistance for stroke survivors who are independent in self-care. I am reluctant to pay a maid service because it would mean I couldn't afford to have my hair cut and colored at an upscale salon. My current strategy is to clean my house as best as I can. Cleaning varies from easy to difficult.

Kitchen clean-up. Washing dishes turned out to be easy. Have I said how much I love my dishwasher? Every stroke survivor needs one. I have a double sink so I put a dish drainer in the sink closest to the dishwasher to collect dirty dishes and act as a staging area. This makes loading the dishwasher easy and fast. It takes me ten minutes to get the dirty dishes out of sight. If you want to hand wash a single dish, you need something to hold the dish still so it won't spin around in the sink as you scrub it. Put an "octopus pad" under the dish. These round rubber pads have little suction cups on both sides. They used to be readily available, but I could find them only at www.sammonspreston.com. Even with these suction pads, washing dishes one-handed is slow. You'll be spending a significant part of your day washing dishes if you don't have a dishwasher.

Low-tech solutions make kitchen clean-up easy. Fill a liquid soap dispenser with dishwashing detergent. Turn the nozzle so it faces away from you and can catch the liquid soap in your cupped fingers as you push down on the pump with your palm (the **backwards rule**). It's hard to tear off a paper towel one-handed without unrolling several sheets when the roll is on an overhead towel rack. Instead, store the roll of paper towels vertically on the counter so you can pick it up and hold it against your stomach while tearing off a sheet. It's easier to get lids on and off of cheap disposable storage containers than expensive ones, like Tupperware. To store food in a zip-lock bag, line a measuring cup with a zip-lock bag. Put your hand inside the bag and stuff the bag into the measuring cup. Work your hand back out without removing the bag and work the sides of the zip-lock bag over the sides of the cup. When the bag is half full, pull the bag out of the cup. The weight of the food will keep the bag open as you finish filling it.

Taking out the garbage is relatively easy. It isn't what I wanted to do after my stroke, but kitchen garbage can get ripe quickly. Taking out the garbage doesn't lend itself to a family member dropping by in a few days to take care of it. Skip this topic if you do not have the following skills. Taking out the garbage is not safe unless you (1) can walk up and down stairs independently and (2) can walk outdoors for a short distance without a cane so you don't lean on the garbage because you have poor **balance**.

I walk well enough to lift a full garbage bag out of the container by the drawstrings without losing my balance. I place the bag on the seat of a nearby kitchen chair so I don't have to bend down to tie the strings. Make sure the drawstring is pulled tight and make a tight knot using your teeth and sound hand. Put a new bag in the garbage container by trapping one side over the rim with your hemiplegic hand and stretching the other side of the bag over the rim with your sound hand. Hefty makes a kitchen garbage bag called "The Gripper" with an elasticized draw string that doesn't slip off the rim when you let go.

Transport the full garbage bag to the door with a **rolling cart**. I kick the tightly closed garbage bag down the stairs instead of carrying it and keep my outside garbage can nearby by placing it behind my front steps. I live next to a wooded area that has raccoons, so I can't leave my garbage can unlocked. To take the cover off the garbage can, I lean on the cover with my hemiplegic elbow and unlock the lid with my sound hand. To get the garbage can to the curb, I push it ahead of me by turning the wheels to the *front* so the back half slides on the concrete (the **backwards rule**). Sliding gradually wears out the bottom of the can, but replacing a garbage can every two or three years is far cheaper than a trip to the emergency room.

Bathroom clean-up. The only thing that makes cleaning the toilet a challenge is opening the childproof cap on the toilet bowl cleaner with one hand. Clorox saves the day. The cap of a Clorox container of toilet bowl cleaner is never removed. Twist the cap slightly to raise it a fraction of an inch to let the liquid flow through the spout. Have someone untwist the cap if it isn't safe for you to lean forward in sitting, hold the bottle between your feet, and push down as you untwist the cap with your sound hand. When you are finished, don't twist the cap down tight so it is easy to open the next time. Not closing the cap tightly probably causes the liquid to dry out faster, but the way I look at it, thicker liquid clings to the sides of the toilet bowl better.

Cleaning the shower is easy if you cheat. It is unsafe to lean over to scrub the shower by hand. SC Johnson makes a dispenser that automatically sprays the shower every day with Scrubbing Bubbles and cleans by letting the solution slide down the walls. I don't use the automatic dispenser because I don't want residue building up on the seat of my shower chair and the nylon-net poof and back scrubber I leave hanging in the shower, but it gave me an idea. I clean my shower by using a spray can of Scrubbing Bubbles and coming back later to hose down the walls with my adapted shower hose. It helps that I use shower gel. A liquid form of soap doesn't leave the soap scum associated with hard bars of soap. I've stopped feeling guilty about not scrubbing my shower by hand because I'm doing more to clean my shower than some able-bodied people.

Floors and carpets. Cleaning a floor is a challenge. Skip this topic if you do not have the following skill. Cleaning the kitchen and bathroom floor is not safe unless you can walk without using a walker or cane indoors.

Preparing the floor by sweeping it with a broom is difficult when you don't have good movement in both arms and hands. It's easier to vacuum linoleum floors with a stick vacuum. This type of vacuum is lightweight and has a rechargeable battery instead of a cord. Using a cordless stick vacuum is much safer than wrestling with the long hose and cord of a canister vacuum. I found one at a local vacuum cleaner store. Stick vacuums are sold on the Internet, but I wanted to make sure I could empty the container that collects the debris and remove the rechargeable battery. Shopping at a vacuum cleaner store was more expensive, but the sales person was very nice about showing me how to perform these functions and letting me try them myself before I bought the vacuum.

Moving chairs out of the way is a difficult part of washing the floor, so I leave most of my dining room chairs lined up against one wall until company comes. No one walks along this wall so I cheat and just vacuum the floor under this line of chairs. The dirtiest part of the floor is in the food preparation area, like in front of the stove, sink, and refrigerator.

For safety, I wash linoleum floors while standing using a Swiffer WetJet. A container of washing fluid is attached to the handle. The container is easy to install and remove one-handed. A push button on the handle sprays the liquid. A disposable cleaning pad is held in place by Velcro strips and traps the dirty cleaning solution behind a one-way barrier, just like a disposable diaper. The swivel head makes it easy to get into corners. The only disadvantage of the Swiffer WetJet is that small pieces of debris gradually pile up along the baseboards, so a periodic cleaning by an able-bodied person is recommended.

I bought a lightweight steam floor cleaner, but it was too difficult for me to handle. Once the cleaning head becomes damp, it creates a lot of resistance for someone with a stroke. The TV commercial uses long shots while the actors chat and hold a steam cleaner with no cord attached. The commercial switches to close-ups when actual cleaning is done and shows the user walking forwards in a long straight line. However, the steam cleaner lacks an on-off button so if you don't want to pull the plug by walking on your wet floor when you are finished, you have to start as far away as you can get from the electrical outlet and back up. Walking backwards while you maneuver around furniture is difficult after a stroke. You have to rewind the cord quickly each time you back up so the hot steam doesn't damage the floor because you've left the cleaner in one place too long. The cord was not long enough to clean my whole kitchen so I had to use a heavy-duty extension cord, which added to the weight.

Vacuuming is the most difficult cleaning task I do because it requires both good **balance** and good **endurance**. Skip this topic if you do not have the following skills. Vacuuming is not safe unless you (1) can use your hemiplegic hand to hold the cord away from your body so your feet won't get tangled in the cord and (2) can step over the cord without using a cane.

A vacuum cleaner is heavy enough to help me keep my balance, but the weight tires me out. It took five months before I could vacuum three rooms in one day without stopping to rest. Two strategies make vacuuming easier. First, I bought a lighter vacuum cleaner that is less tiring to push around. It's a Hoover model called the Tempo. The Tempo weighs eighteen pounds instead of the usual twenty-two to twenty-five pounds. Second, I finally accepted that I have to vacuum very slowly. Slowing down reduces the other tiring aspect of vacuuming which is the non-stop change of direction. A self-propelled vacuum doesn't eliminate this problem. A self-propelled vacuum really flies when you pull on the handle. This would speed up how fast I would have to step forward and back up.

Small Tasks that Fall through the Cracks

Small tasks fall through the cracks because they come up only once in a while and take very little time. My neighbor Raffeala **volunteered** to keep an extra key to my house in case I get locked out. She collects my mail when I go away and brings my empty garbage can in from the curb if she goes out before I do. Raffaela lends me her husband once every three or four months to do small chores. Mike replaces batteries in my smoke alarms, replaces burnt-out light bulbs in ceiling lights, tightens loose screws, puts together purchases that have to be assembled, and sets up my artificial Christmas tree.

Helping with small homecare tasks you know how to do, like changing a light bulb, can **prevent a fall** and help a stroke survivor stay in his or her home. These small tasks are the kind of thing you can't hire people to do. If you don't have helpful neighbors as I do, try calling your church. These small tasks might be a good **volunteer** project for the teen group to take on. It helps to be efficient when asking for this kind of sporadic help. I save up chores that can wait and make a list that people can do in one visit instead of calling them repeatedly to do two-minute tasks.

The Bottom Line

The home health OT who treated me after my first stroke didn't address homecare issues. In his defense, I was glad to have him concentrate on my hemiplegic arm and hand because I was too exhausted to do housework. When I left my wheelchair at the hospital, it took me two months to develop the **endurance** I needed to walk everywhere indoors. By the time I had the endurance and balance to think about homecare tasks, my home health benefits were exhausted. You may regain endurance more quickly than I did so you may be able to start homecare training sooner.

If low endurance slows your progress, you may be eligible for homecare training even if your home health benefits are used up. Medicare provision 220.1.4 allows outpatient departments to treat clients who are well enough to travel but who need to learn homecare in a familiar environment (CMS, 2007). An innovative OT persuaded a traditional outpatient department to send its therapists into homes so they could see that providing this service is both practical and successful (Toto, 2008). It's safer to explore your homecare interests if you have a therapist by your side who can anticipate problems and help you succeed.

Your doctor will write a general prescription, like "improve safety during homecare tasks." Insurance companies pay attention when you raise safety issues. Yet I don't recommend this shotgun approach when you see the OT. Congress threatens every year to stop allowing exceptions to the $1,800 cap on Medicare reimbursement for outpatient OT. Tell the OT you want to know how safe you are with homecare tasks you are interested in and ask the OT to address these specific concerns.

The homecare tasks you are willing and able to do depend on what kind of stroke you had and on what ADL tasks you like to do. I had to iron sheets for a family of seven in the days before permanent press so a therapist had better not try to teach me to iron one-handed. I hope my descriptions make it clear which homecare tasks are easier to do safely. Even if you do only a little bit of homecare, it can take pressure off of your caregivers. Doing simple tasks, like answering the phone, means the people caring for you can do more activities without being interrupted and worry less when they run errands.

If homecare is difficult for you, it's a temptation to micromanage how other people do it for you. Because stroke survivors have done homecare for years, we have developed our own ways of doing things that are familiar and comforting. For example, after I got married my mother criticized the way I loaded her dishwasher when I came over for dinner. She must have wanted my help because she stopped making remarks about where I placed the dishes in the rack. People are going to stop **volunteering** to help us stay in our homes if we insist they do everything the way we used to do it.

When taking care of myself gets to be too much for me, I hope to go to assisted living. While this setting will give me more freedom than a nursing home, I still won't be able to tell the staff they have to wash my underwear in Ivory Flakes. It will be difficult to express my gratitude while I am mourning the loss of my home. I hope I will learn to be grateful when the clean clothes I get back from the laundry are my own.

References

Centers for Medicare & Medicaid Services, (2007). *Medicare benefit policy manual*. Chapter 15: Covered medical and other health services. Retrieved February 17, 2008 from http://www.cms.hhs.gov/manuals.

Toto, P. (2008). The impact of context: OT services in the home and community. *OT Practice*, May 12, 17-21.

CHAPTER 6

ADVANCED ADLs IN THE COMMUNITY

Except for gait training and driver education, you're on your own when it comes to regaining independence in advanced Activities of Daily Living (ADLs) in the community. Insurance companies don't pay therapists to teach clients how to maneuver in restaurants or get on airplanes. You have to do the legwork to find out if you are eligible for community services, like Paratransit. Social workers in your rehab hospital don't know the criteria that qualify you for community services because the criteria vary by county. I found that websites for county and state services are vague or out of date in my area. Talking to a person about my situation made it easier to get specific information about what services I qualified for. Contact your county's Council on Aging, which has lots of information about services for the disabled, and the National Council on Independent Living (see Appendix C). Don't assume that being homebound is inevitable. Don't assume you will never eat out or travel again. This chapter illustrates how much mobility stroke survivors can regain in their communities.

Keys, Money, and Purses Come First

The first thing you have to do to get out of your house is lock your front door. Digging for a key is nerve-wracking after you have a stroke. My days of fishing through a purse or sorting through a full ring of keys to find my house key are over. Even though I have a purse that hangs across my torso by a long strap, it takes two hands to dig through a purse; one hand to hold the objects aside so I can see and the other hand to dig around for the key.

One way to quickly lock your front door is to keep your house key on a stretchy plastic coil that clips onto your purse. Or attach your house key to a plastic coil that stretches over your wrist and fits in your pants pocket. This wrist coil does double duty. It makes it easier to locate the key in your pocket by feel and allows you to put the key around your wrist when you want to pick up an object. I had a house key fall underneath my stairs when I set it on a flat surface while I

106

opened the screen door. It is also nerve-wracking to unlock a door without adequate lighting. I had an electrician install a motion-sensitive porch light that goes on as I approach the house. I feel safe because I can get into my house quickly and safely. It was money well spent.

Once you're out of the house, you have to manage your wallet and purse. People with two hands can fumble through a purse to find something, but a stroke makes this frustrating. Before each trip, place objects you will need for a particular trip in your wallet or in an accessible place in your purse. Examples include taking an ATM card when you go to the bank and a library card when you go to the library to check out a book or DVD. The days of carrying every credit card I own are over. My Visa card stays in a zippered compartment where it's safe and can be quickly retrieved and put away. Other credit cards come out of my desk only for special trips. When you get home, take objects you no longer need out of your wallet or purse.

Handling money while shopping is easy. When you are alone in line, you have the luxury of taking your time to fish out the exact change. If there are people behind you in line, I give the cashier more money than the bill requires. When the cashier hands me the change and receipt, I dump them in my pants pocket or purse. I put the change in my wallet after I get home. Not having the people behind me glare at me while I fumble with money is a relief. I put a small piece of clear **Dycem** in my purse or wallet to keep credit card slips from sliding when I sign them. Simple strategies for handling money make it easier to venture into the community. Getting out of the house is supposed to be a treat, not a source of anxiety.

Eating Out Takes Practice

Eating out takes planning, but it gives me a chance to visit with family and friends, to eat cuisine I don't know how to cook, and freedom from cooking. I feel nervous the first time I tackle a new dining venue, but I also feel pampered. I was the oldest girl in a family of seven, so mealtime meant a lot of work when I was growing up. If you want to go to an unfamiliar restaurant, calling before you go may make you less anxious. Do they have (a) handicapped parking, (b) stairs or a ramp, (c) hand railings on both sides, (d) **wheelchair** seating, and (e) wheelchair-accessible bathrooms? If you love to eat out, don't give up.

My first dining experience took place while I was still in rehab. My recreational therapist took me to an ice cream shop. I had transferred out of my wheelchair in the hospital so many times that sliding in and out of the booth was easy. What I wasn't prepared for was how it felt to deal with a stranger's reaction to me in a wheelchair. When I rolled up to pay the bill, the cashier looked at my therapist when I tried to hand her the bill and my money. Interacting with strangers who are standing while you are sitting in a wheelchair puts you at a social disadvantage. Having someone to whom I had spoken avoid eye contact made me feel awful. It was humiliating to be a disembodied voice on the other side of a counter. When I stood up, she looked startled. I had her attention once our eyes were on the same level. Even if the person accompanying you has to tell the waitress what you want, don't look down and let other people get away with not acknowledging you by avoiding eye contact.

Different dining environments create different mobility challenges. Going to breakfast at a crowded café with my friends requires slow, careful maneuvering while walking between closely placed tables and chairs. This is another instance where walking in straight lines with a PT doesn't prepare you for the community. The first time I went to a private dinner party that was served buffet style, I slid my plate along the table but had to have someone **transport** it to my seat. I found an end table to set my plate on because I can't juggle it on my lap anymore. I transferred this strategy to a salad bar. You can place the plate at different points along the front of a salad bar. It's a treat to take your time to make your own selections. If it is unsafe for you to walk short distances without a cane, ask a companion to carry your plate to the table.

Cutting food requires its own strategies. I keep a rocker knife in my purse so I can cut food one-handed. The knife is hard to get in and out of my purse because it is so long. Someone needs to invent a folding rocker knife. I wash the dirty knife when I get home, put it in a new zip-lock bag, and put it back in my purse for next time. Otherwise I have to remember to take a rocker knife out of the drawer each time I eat out. Rocker knives are relatively dull, so I don't order dense food like steak or slippery food like chicken on the bone. You may decide to order these foods if you don't feel self-conscious about having someone cut your food into bite-size pieces. Occasionally, a plate won't stay still when I cut food so I slip the small rectangle of clear **Dycem** I carry in my purse under my plate. Even a napkin under a plate may provide enough friction to hold the plate still.

I don't go to the bathroom when I eat out if I can help it, but sometimes Mother Nature insists. To keep from having to sit on **public toilet** seats, I fold over several layers of toilet paper and drape the paper perpendicular to the toilet seat. Each side of the seat has its own pile. The weight of the paper draped over the sides of the seat keeps the paper still. Fortunately, more and more bathrooms in my area are stocked with disposable paper toilet seat covers, which are easier to handle. Finally, it's vital to have a wad of **toilet paper** in your hand before you sit down. The toilet paper dispenser is not always on the wall closest to you while you are sitting on the toilet. You don't want to stand up with your pants around your ankles while you search for the end of the roll.

Paratransit Really Works

Daytime appointments can place a burden on your support system. Paratransit is an invaluable service because many stroke survivors need to go places during working hours, like outpatient therapy, the brace man, and the dentist. Employers grant family leave when a health crisis first occurs, but then they expect the problem to go away. A family member who is the main source of income and health benefits can't jeopardize his or her job by repeatedly asking for time off during the day. Even if your family lives close by, consider using Paratransit services for some trips during the day.

While living with my friend, I found that most of the places I needed to go were in the next county where I used to live. This meant I couldn't use *county* Paratransit services because this service doesn't cross county lines. However, a county staff member told me about the *state* Paratransit system. Here is an example of a restriction that can limit your eligibility. I have to live no more than seven-tenths of a mile from an existing bus or train route to qualify for state Paratransit services.

It's not enough to give Paratransit your diagnosis in order to qualify for the service. You have to explain how your disability makes it impossible for you to take public transportation. After a one-hour interview, I qualified for Paratransit services because I need two accommodations. The drivers accommodate my difficulty with **multitasking** while I'm standing. They give me all the time I need to put my **cane** and packages down to free my hands to get the exact change out of my purse and visually locate an empty seat. They also accommodate my poor **balance** by making sure the vehicle doesn't move until I'm seated with my seatbelt buckled. Be prepared to explain specific accommodations you need if you apply for Paratransit services.

I'm lucky to live in a densely populated area that provides Paratransit services that run the same hours as buses and trains. The cost for each trip is based on what it would cost me to take the same trip on public transportation (e.g., $1.10 one-way). I have to have exact change, but the person who schedules my trip tells me how much the fare will be. This gives me the opportunity to put my fare in a pocket or an envelope that I hand to the driver.

A computer printout helps me manage the information that Paratransit requires when I make a reservation. Paratransit must have the street address, town, and phone number for every destination. I print out an updated copy of this information on a sheet of paper that I carry in my purse or wallet. It helps to carry a small calendar to write down the destinations, pick-up and return times, and the fare that varies for each trip. You can take my money, but leave my Paratransit calendar.

Putting the drivers' names and a brief description of each person on my list is useful. Paratransit staff don't get paid a big salary. The person that plans their route is in another part of the state and may plan a tour that is impossible. Sometimes drivers have to cut out their lunch breaks to stay on schedule. I show my appreciation and respect for these underpaid staff by remembering their names and saying thank you every time I use this service. A number of drivers are very friendly and I look forward to chatting with them on each trip.

As wonderful as they are, my Paratransit services have seven limitations. First, Paratransit in my state is a "curb-to-curb" service. This means you or a caretaker has to get you out of your house and to the curb and then from the curb back into your house. Second, you have to phone twenty-four hours in advance to schedule a ride, so this service is not designed to handle emergencies. Third, my Paratransit's shortest turn-around time is an hour and a half. If I want to do one thing like mail a package, the driver won't wait for me and take me home. I have to wait to be picked up by a second bus.

Fourth, my Paratransit service has a two-bag limit and doesn't allow staff to carry packages for me. If you are in a wheelchair, the driver will put your packages on the lift with you, but that's it. I walk onto the bus so I have to get my bags on and off the bus and get them into my house. This doesn't allow me to shop for a lot of items in one run.

The fifth limitation is the forty-minute window at both ends of the trip. For instance, if I ask to be picked up at 10:00 a.m., the actual pick-up time can occur anytime between 9:40 and 10:20. I may go directly to my destination or I may ride for up to an hour if two to three other people are on my tour. The drop-off order is determined by who got on first. Unless my destination is on the way to someone else's, I may get off last so the person who got on first won't be late for his or her appointment. The company gets fined every time a client is late.

The sixth limitation is that the driver will wait only five minutes after he pulls up. Therapy appointments usually run like clockwork and are a good match for this short time limit. However, my Paratransit can't deal with appointments that consistently run late, like doctors' appointments. I use a local medical transport company that is free if their services are requested by a medical professional. The office staff call to set up the trip and the company calls me to confirm the pick-up time. When my medical appointment is over, the office staff calls the company to come pick me up.

The seventh limitation is that you are always on the Paratransit clock. One day, I got so involved while shopping that I missed my pick-up. This is called a "No Show." I had to wait an hour for another bus driver to change his route to pick me up. A few days later, I got a warning letter telling me that if I had three no-shows in a thirty-day period, my privileges would be revoked. Now I always keep track of the time when I go shopping with Paratransit.

This seventh limitation means Paratransit isn't suited to social activities where you want to relax. A small, rotating group of friends took turns transporting me to social activities until I could drive. They took me to the breakfast club we attend once a week. They transported me to dinner parties so my host didn't have to worry about my showing up forty minutes early or having to walk out the door before dessert was served. If my friends couldn't pick me up they said no, so I didn't worry too much about imposing. Paratransit provided the vast majority of my other rides, so I asked my friends for a ride only to social activities.

Combining several Paratransit services and friends who drove me places was a good mix. Consider using a variety of transportation solutions instead of relying on one person to drive you everywhere. Another Paratransit service that is better suited to grocery shopping is described in the next section.

Shopping with Paratransit

If you drive, have family nearby, or can afford to have groceries delivered, you may not have to shop with Paratransit. However, going into an institution is a high price to pay because you don't have someone to pick up a prescription or buy a carton of milk. When I was able-bodied, I shopped at the end of my commute from work, so I was amazed to learn how many times Americans drive to a store. If you've always had a car, it's hard to appreciate that shopping is a part-time job we embed in our busy schedules.

One alternative is to buy groceries through a professional shopping service. I found a local company that shops for clients at the most expensive grocery store in my area. Before gasoline prices shot up this service cost $40 a month. This is a luxury I can't afford on a fixed income, although I used it for three months when I came home after my second stroke. This company isn't affiliated with the store so it doesn't have access to a list of the thousands of items available at the store. Instead of shopping from a posted list, I had to send the company an e-mail listing everything I wanted. My list had to be very specific, like Post Shredded Wheat 'n Bran Spoon Sized. Think about how many kinds of shredded wheat cereal a professional shopper has to choose from. The one thing that surprised me about the male shoppers is that they always picked out flawless fresh fruits and vegetables.

If you can't afford to pay a professional shopper, Paratransit may be the answer to your prayers. However, transporting my purchases was a challenge that took trial-and-error to figure out. Transferring items to a backpack before I left the store was tiring and frustrating. I felt self-conscious as I stood at the end of an unused cash register line to pack and repack a large load to make everything fit so the zipper would close. A fully loaded backpack can be difficult to swing onto your shoulders and <u>make you unsafe</u> because it challenges your **balance**. My solution was to split my purchases between a backpack and a small, light **folding cart** that holds one paper bag's worth of purchases. Dozens of companies sell these small carts on the Internet. Google "folding grocery carts." I put a few heavy items in the backpack so I can carry them close to my body and put light, bulky items in the cart, which makes it easier to lift up the bus steps.

There are four constraints when you use a small folding cart. First, it <u>must be safe for you</u> to lift the light cart into the store's shopping cart. Second, you have to limit your purchases to what fits in the child seat of the shopping cart, although what fits in the child seat is remarkable. Third, you may have to get the cart on the Paratransit bus yourself. I can lift the cart up to the second step of the Paratransit bus. The driver can reach over and hold the handle of the cart until I get up the steps because Paratransit mini-buses are narrower than a regular bus. Then I lean down to pull the cart up the last step. If you don't have good standing **balance**, leaning over even this slight amount <u>may not be safe for you</u>. The last constraint is getting the cart up the stairs to the front door of your house. I found a method that is suitable for short people and shallow steps (short from front to back). When I asked a co-worker to try my method, <u>she felt unsafe</u> because she is taller and the stairs she was using were deeper than mine at home.

If getting purchases on and off a Paratransit bus <u>isn't realistic for you</u>, investigate senior citizens' services for your county. I saw senior citizens being picked up twice a week in my subdivision so on a whim I called my township. I'm not a senior citizen, but because I am disabled I was allowed to ride the bus on its regular Tuesday run. I rode with the seniors to the senior citizen center and then the bus driver took me to the grocery store. This service has a three-bag limit and runs only from 10:00 to 2:30, Monday through Friday. However, it is a "door-to-door" service. The drivers are used to carrying packages for frail, elderly clients and escorting them and their purchases to the front door of their homes.

Using the senior citizens' bus allowed me to go grocery shopping once a week because I could use a heavier (15-pound) **folding cart** that holds two full bags of groceries. I didn't have to lift this heavier cart into the store's grocery cart because I could push and steer this taller and more stable folding cart with both hands. I hung a soft nylon cooler (big enough for 24 beer cans) by its shoulder strap on the front end of my cart. This gave me a place to put meat and frozen food. When I emptied this cooler at the checkout lane, all my cold foods were together. The cashiers would put the cold food into the cooler instead of a grocery bag and most were kind enough to zip it closed for me. At the checkout lane, I put two empty paper bags in my folding cart, filled the bags with groceries, and plopped the nylon cooler on top. The senior citizen bus driver lifted this heavily loaded cart on and off the bus, carried it up my front steps, and brought it inside while I held the door open.

Even these adapted procedures weren't enough to meet non-food needs, like buying bulky paper towels and heavy containers of laundry detergent. I didn't purchase these household goods in the grocery shop because I used the space in my cart for food. Until I could drive, a friend **volunteered** every six months to pick me up at the store after I shopped for a big order, bring me home, and help me get my purchases into the house. I can buy in bulk because I have a lot of storage space at home.

Despite the limitations, I would have had to enter an institution without Paratransit services. It is a wise use of public funds that gives people independence without costing the thousands of dollars that institutional care requires. I am grateful to have this resource and suggest that you look into what is available in your area. Shopping is one of the biggest obstacles to staying in your own home.

Shopping for Clothes is Like Going to War

I buy a lot of things online, but clothing isn't one of them. I am one size on top and another size on the bottom, so I have to try on a lot of outfits to find one that fits. I am also particular about how comfortable a garment feels. Clothing costs too much to pay for outfits that don't feel good. When I shop for clothes, I think like a general who is going to war. A general relies on good reconnaissance and organization. You may think this analogy is over the top, but I may change your mind.

On Day 1, if you don't know what floor the clothing department is on, call the store to find out so you can park on the same level. If you plan to shop at more than one store, your first assignment for Day 1 is to find out if clothing departments in different stores are located on different levels. If they are, scout out the location of elevators if you need them. The elevators aren't likely to be conveniently located, so finding them on Day 1 will let you know to set aside extra time when you come back to make your purchases.

The second assignment for Day 1 is finding clothes that you like. Clothing is subdivided by fashion designer. This means that one type of garment, like pants, can be spread across the entire clothing department. I can walk in a straight line for a quarter of a mile without sitting down to rest, but shopping wears me out quickly because it requires non-stop turning. You have to turn to walk around racks of clothing and turn to look at each display you are interested in. Every time I turn towards my sound left side, my hemiplegic right leg flies out to the side. I have to expend extra energy to bring it back in front of my body before I take my next step. After you have located elevators, found clothes you like, and located the dressing rooms, go home and rest. I don't remember every piece of clothing I liked, but I can eliminate a large portion of the store. Think like a general who scouts out the terrain before going to battle.

On Day 2, wear clothes that are easy to take off and put on. I wear pants with an elastic waistband and a loose-fitting pullover top. If

I'm shopping for a few items, I go alone and bring my small **folding cart** to drape the clothes over as I make my selections. If you need a lot of clothes, it's best if someone accompanies you to the store. Your companion can carry the clothes you've selected to the dressing room.

When you get to the dressing room, it helps to hang the clothes up in a particular order. Hang up outfits that have tops last so they are on top of the stack and you can try them on first. Even though I dress myself every day, repeatedly donning clothes makes me sweat because I am working so hard. It's easier to get tops on and off when my back is dry. I throw each garment over my cart after I take it off. I need to sit and rest when I'm finished trying on clothes, so I use this rest period to rehang the garments or let my companion do it. I can rehang pants and skirts by laying them on my lap. My hemiplegic hand holds the garment still while my sound hand brings the opened clips to the clothes (the **backwards rule**). Like a general who moves his troops around, you've got to figure out how to move all those garments around. I go to war when I'm shopping for clothes and I win.

Good Timing is Free

Good timing makes getting around your community easier. Don't go grocery shopping at 5:00 p.m. when everyone gets off from work. Don't go to the movies on Friday night when the new movies come out. Big crowds were exciting when I was young, but even before my stroke I had a "been there, done that" attitude toward crowds. Adults who work and escort children to all their activities don't get to choose when to go out, but good timing is a strategy you can use when you're retired or disabled.

So what does going out at a less crowded time get you? There are fewer maniacs trying to run you off the road when they become enraged by people who are driving the speed limit. You are more likely to find a handicapped parking space. Once you get to the mall, there is less foot traffic. This creates bigger spaces between people so you have more room to maneuver. Maneuvering in a densely packed crowd with a **cane** is tricky. It sticks out six to eight inches from your body and violates the social agreement that people in a crowd are allowed to pass shoulder to shoulder. When a mall is crowded, people have gotten so close to me that I've had to stop walking and pull my cane in to my side to keep from tripping them. Fewer people also means you have fewer distracted people who step into your path. I can stop suddenly these days but still can't step sideways quickly to avoid a collision. Fewer people means more empty chairs and benches if you need to sit down and rest. Store clerks may even be more helpful because they are less rushed and tired. At least checkout lines are shorter.

Maneuvering in Crowds that Sit Down

Because I love to go to movies, I discovered there are safe ways to maneuver in crowds who are sitting down. My best tip is to arrive early and leave late by waiting for the crowd to leave. Arriving early means (a) the house lights are on so you can see, (b) you don't have a lot of people coming up behind you when you are navigating stairs or a sloping floor, and (c) you don't have to stumble past seated people to get to a seat. The best place to sit is in the center of a row. This sounds counterintuitive, but I made the mistake of reserving an aisle seat at a concert and found myself constantly standing up to let people in and out of my row. The best place to stow your **cane** is on the floor under the seat, parallel to your row. This keeps it out of the way so people won't knock it over or trip over it.

If you can walk up and down stairs, you have more seating choices as long as you plan ahead. Movie theaters put handicapped seating in the front of the theater where you go deaf and get a headache from constantly turning your head from side to side to see the action. Fortunately, movie theaters usually have handrails on both sides. To keep the railing on your sound side, walk up one side and down the other. For safety, have someone assist you when you make the transition onto the stairs. You will have to take one or two steps before you can grab the handrail and again when you let go of the handrail to step into the aisle you've selected. Older venues that host plays and concerts often don't have handrails because they were built years ago. Call the box office and inquire about elevators and railings before you reserve a seat that is not on the main floor.

Day-long events where people are standing, like museum exhibits, craft fairs, dog shows, and store windows decorated for the holidays, are more of a challenge than crowds that sit down. If you arrive just before opening or during the last two hours of the event, there are fewer people, more parking spaces, and more places to sit. Of course, this time restriction means not being able to see everything, but in my opinion it beats turning into a couch potato and giving up lifelong forms of recreation. Try going with an able-bodied senior citizen or parents with young children who are used to accommodating people who tire quickly. Getting a stroke survivor out of the house for a few hours of fun is a great gift. It's a great way to **volunteer** without taking up your whole day.

I don't go to *time-limited* events where people are standing, like a parade. I tried going to a historic re-enactment but felt ill at ease. When something exciting happened, people leaned to the left or right to get a better view, which meant I was repeatedly jostled. This is normal crowd behavior that I can't tolerate any more. An outdoor event like a parade also means standing for a long time, which I can't do anymore either. However, an outdoor concert where everyone brings lawn chairs may be possible if the people you go with are willing to wait for the crowd to thin out so you don't get trampled by the first rush of people. Not being able to go to time-limited events makes holidays lonely for stroke survivors.

My **balance** isn't good enough to attend events where people are expected to mingle while standing. For example, I don't get in line to shake my pastor's hand after church. Holding my **cane** in my hemiplegic hand so I can shake hands with my sound hand, trying not to bump into the people ahead of me in line, and talking are too many things for me to manage at one time. I'm more tolerant of children who don't watch where they are going now that I know how many skills it takes to maneuver in a crowd. Processing local information, like managing your body and responding to what the person in front of you is doing, while also keeping track of your progress toward a distant target is a lot to handle when you are in a crowd.

If your balance is better than mine, it may be easier for you to maneuver through a crowd. People who don't need a **cane**, **walker**, or **wheelchair** are less dependent on strangers to anticipate their needs and give them special consideration. On the other hand, if you don't feel safe walking in a crowd, it would be ideal if your home health PT met you at a store or the mall to show you how to navigate safely through a <u>sparse crowd on a weekday</u>. You don't have to be homebound if you go out at the right time in the right kind of crowd.

Americans Love to Drive

I'm proud of being able to care for my home again, but being a homemaker isn't enough for me. I have friends who spend hours creating exquisite home décors and cooking gourmet meals, but these home-based activities require talents that I lack. My talented friends showed me there is another level of homemaking that people other than Martha Stewart enjoy. I don't enjoy cooking and decorating my home because I have to struggle for every success. I need a car to express my talents. I wanted to return to part-time teaching at my old job at a university fifty miles away.

With medical bills coming in, my first concern about driver training was cost. Health insurance doesn't pay for it. If you have the potential to return to work, see if vocational training will pay part of the cost of your driver education. I didn't qualify for this assistance because the paid sick leave I received after my stroke put me over the financial cutoff. However, I valued driving so much that I set aside money in my budget to pay for this service. I was able to pay off the bill gradually at $100 a month.

The training begins. The rehab facility where I was an inpatient has a certified driving instructor. Carrie is an OT with advanced driver training certification, clinical experience, and the equipment I needed to learn adapted driving. She told me to put my request in as soon as possible. There aren't enough OTs who specialize in driving training, so there is a waiting list. I was lucky. I had to wait only two months. I had to bring a written referral for driving training from my doctor to my first appointment. During the first session, she checked visual-perceptual skills, like my peripheral vision, and tested safety awareness by having me analyze various driving scenarios. I was fortunate because I don't have significant perceptual-cognitive deficits from my brainstem stroke.

After I passed the paper-and-pencil tests, Carrie took me out on the road. The training car has a kill switch that allowed her to turn off the engine immediately and an extra brake pedal on the passenger side that allowed her to stop the car. The car modifications Carrie chose for me were a spinner knob that attaches to the steering wheel and a gas pedal extender. The extender puts a gas pedal on the left where my sound left foot can reach it and has a rigid cover in front of the actual accelerator where I rest my hemiplegic foot. This extension puts the gas pedal to the *left* of the brake pedal. Oy!

At first, I was distracted because I had to constantly remind myself that the pedal positions were switched. I had to feel for the two pedals because I couldn't afford to take my eyes off the road to look down to find them. It took about two hours of driving to give me enough confidence to believe that I could learn new habits after driving for thirty-eight years. Of course, in a two-hour lesson, I used this new pedal configuration dozens of time. What really surprised me was the carry-over. My body remembered what I had learned in one session and applied it to the next.

Carrie started my training by driving the car to a deserted parking lot where there weren't any cars. This location helped me relax because it minimized the consequences of my errors. I could take out a tree but not kill a person. She had me practice turning left and right by driving around the parking lot in both directions. After that was going well, she had me practice pulling into a parking space and backing out. Then Carrie graduated me to driving on the road. She knew the area well and gradually directed me to more congested areas as I improved. She used the following progression over six lessons: (1) driving on side streets with no traffic, (2) on side streets with some traffic, (3) on busy two-lane streets, (4) on the interstate, and finally (5) in an intense downtown center with lots of pedestrians, cars, and businesses.

Finding out that Carrie could anticipate my errors gave me confidence. For instance, she knew that clients often have trouble doing a K-turn to completely turn a car around. This maneuver requires shifting gears from reverse to first gear and back again. Carrie had her hand on the kill switch before I began so she was able to stop the car when I panicked before I drove the car up onto someone's lawn.

There were a few problems I didn't anticipate. At first, my stiff trunk made it hard to turn and look over my left shoulder. Able-bodied people can put both hands on the steering wheel to keep their upper body still as they turn around to look behind them. I was also surprised by how much abdominal strength it takes to turn a car with one hand on the spinner knob. I often grunt when turning a corner. Finally, I had forgotten how tiring driving is. Making constant decisions in traffic is mentally exhausting. Carrie had me back in the hospital parking lot by the time my **endurance** was running low.

My driving lesson always ended in a special area of the hospital parking lot where Carrie had set up cones to simulate a parallel parking situation. This practice space is identical to the space the Division of Motor Vehicles (DMV) has on its on-the-road test track. Carrie's patience was phenomenal because she knew the DMV passes only drivers who parallel park without so much as touching the curb with a wheel. Even though I was a good parallel parker before my stroke, I had to practice parallel parking ten to fifteen times every session.

After I parked perfectly six times in a row, Carrie said I was ready for the on-the-road test at the DMV. She knows this course well and prepared me for every part of the test. She didn't take me to be tested until she was sure I was ready, so I passed the road test on the first try. That was a confidence builder. She even stood in line with me to get my new license. This was helpful because the staff member at the counter tried to make excuses for why she didn't have the authority to give me a license.

After I got my new driver's license, I had to buy a new car. I donated my old car with a stick shift and 160,000 miles on it to a charity. Just days before my stroke, I had obtained a car loan and had test-driven a new Toyota, so I had already made up my mind about what car I wanted to buy. Toyota and other car manufacturers have a rebate program that reimburses you for car modifications when you purchase a new car. Carrie recommended a business that modifies cars and vans that was five miles from my Toyota dealer. An employee from Accessible Vans picked up my new car and a week later it was ready.

On the road again. I was nervous when a friend took me to pick up my new car because I had to drive home on a multilane highway without my therapist. On the way home I discovered something that helped me relax immediately. There are plenty of trucks and cars in the right-hand lane that are going at or below the speed level. This was a huge surprise. Like so many drivers in frantic New Jersey, I had always rushed everywhere I drove. Driving slowly in the right lane has two advantages. First, my reactions don't have to be as fast because everyone is moving slower. Second, aggressive drivers who try to push you down the road don't have the patience to use the slow lane. I stay in the right lane except when I pass very slow drivers. The only time staying in the right-hand lane doesn't work is when I'm on a six-lane road that has a lot of stores on it. There are so many shoppers pulling in and out of the right lane that I move to the center lane.

Even after my superb training, I was still nervous. Introducing challenges one at a time made it easier to keep my anxiety under control. At first, I drove only (a) in non-rush hour traffic, (b) on local streets, (c) during daylight hours, and (d) for short distances, like five-mile trips. I confined early trips to routes that I knew well. Knowing where every light and left-turn lane is helped me anticipate the moves of other drivers. Over a six-month period, I gradually increased the distance of my trips, drove in rush-hour traffic on local streets, and drove at night on routes I know well. I waited until I was comfortable with each new challenge before I progressed to the next one.

I needed this gradual re-introduction to driving because the size of my new car and the exact location of the spinner knob and gas pedal extension were a little different from the car I had trained on. I also found to my dismay that when I started to relax and pay less attention to my driving, I occasionally stepped on the wrong pedal! Thirty-eight years of stepping on the left-hand pedal to brake reasserted itself and, of course, when I step on the left pedal now the car accelerates. It took three to four months of gently pressing on each pedal to feel what happened to the car before I trusted myself to automatically step on the correct pedal to brake.

I put off interstate driving until last. I knew that driving tight cloverleafs to get on and off an interstate would require sustained upper-body strength. Driving a cloverleaf on or off ramp is like holding a right-hand turn for twenty-five seconds (I actually timed it by counting one-one thousand, etc.). This prolonged turn takes both arm and abdominal strength. Luck was with me the first time I tried it because a big truck got off just before me. The driver behind me was impatient, but he knew I couldn't go faster than the truck. Since that lucky break, I've turned into one of those irritating people who drive cloverleafs as slowly as a truck, which turns out to be the posted speed limit. I drove to work via interstates for eighteen years so I'm not intimidated by quickly accelerating at the end of the on-ramp to blend in with traffic. However, interstate driving may not be safe for you if your prior experience was primarily driving on local streets.

Even with eighteen years of interstate experience, I put off driving on the interstate during rush-hour until last. I had one success and one failure. I do well on the less congested expressways in central Jersey by staying in the slow lane and passing only an occasional slowpoke. In this less intense environment, I don't have to wait long for the congestion to clear before I change lanes. However, driving in north Jersey where commuters are headed for New York City was hair-raising. Staying in the slow right lane didn't protect me from aggressive north Jersey drivers. I drive more defensively than ever and like to stay at least three car lengths from the car in front of me. North Jersey drivers see this open space as an invitation to quickly jump into my lane. By quick I mean pulling diagonally into the space to keep me from speeding up to close the gap. After three drivers swerved into my lane without leaving room for their car to clear the front end of my vehicle, I was shook up. If I hadn't hit my brakes, I would have been in a multi-car accident. Even after two years of driving, I don't trust myself to hit the correct pedal under panic conditions. I avoid the rush hour on congested expressways by driving on them in the middle of the day.

Parking. To get a handicapped parking tag, you need to pick up an application at your local police station in the town where you reside.

Each town has a different form. Your doctor needs to sign the form, so remember to get the form before you see your doctor. The tag won't do you much good in densely populated areas. Handicapped spaces are usually taken where I live unless I go to less popular stores, like Staples.

The time I resent able-bodied drivers who have borrowed a hangtag the most is when I go grocery shopping. Handicapped spaces are wider, so it is easier to load groceries in the car. Having extra space to put the **shopping cart** right next to my car means I can easily place a bag on the backseat. In narrower spaces, I have to carry each bag to the car from a shopping cart that is positioned behind or in front of my car. Easily seventy-five percent of drivers getting out of cars in handicapped parking spaces are in their 40s and 50s with no visible handicap. Are there really that many middle-aged people with crippling lung or heart disease?

Unfortunately, doctors who certify drivers as eligible for a handicapped parking tag have an incentive to give them out. They don't want to alienate a client over a silly thing like not approving a hangtag. We have to find another way to decide who really needs a hang tag. In the meantime, when I get angry I remind myself that the extra walking I am doing is helping me keep my weight down. The people who think they have found a smart parking strategy will get their just rewards. Their laziness puts them at greater risk for high blood pressure and obesity. If I'm really angry, I picture them with crippling arthritis or a stroke. Then I feel bad and try to let go of my anger. There is no point in giving myself a heart attack.

Parking in the summer is complicated by the fact that the sun superheats the spinner knob on my steering wheel. Accordion-type sunshields are a nightmare to put up one-handed. Believe me, I've really tried. As soon as you get one part of the shield up, another part falls out of position. Sunshields that come in two separate parts and resemble the two halves of a giant pair of sunglasses are the only way to go. It takes about ten seconds (honest) to get the two halves up and I succeed on the first try every time. Manufacturers designed this type of sunshield to be twisted so each half can be folded into a circle, but I leave them open and stuff them between the door and the passenger's seat. <u>For safety, make sure</u> the sunshield doesn't obscure the side-view mirror on the passenger's side before you drive off. Throw the sunshields in the back seat when you have a passenger. Read the package instructions to make sure you buy the correct size for your vehicle.

Car maintenance. While the accelerator pedal extension is a blessing, it is also a curse when it comes to car maintenance. Three men who moved my car with the gas pedal extension in place had nervous grins on their faces when they told me what they had done. I've mistakenly stepped on the wrong pedal enough times to know what they did. Mechanics who have to maneuver my car around a crowded parking lot freak me out if they drive with the adapted pedal in place. The only guy I trust to drive my car with the adapted pedal in place is the mechanic who changes my oil. Since it's a small gas station, I can leave my car parked close to the bay door. He drives the car a short distance by putting the car in gear and letting the automatic transmission roll the car into the bay without touching the accelerator pedal.

For other types of maintenance, I remove the adapted gas pedal myself because auto mechanics don't listen to handicapped women. It has a quick-release mechanism: (1) pull up a ring to release the mechanism and (2) pull out the whole unit while holding the pin in the up position. I remove the adapted pedal with help from a long-handled reacher I keep in the trunk of my car. Because I don't do this task regularly, it takes two or three tries. It's less stressful if I park where there is no traffic and can take my time. This procedure takes patience and persistence, but it keeps my blood pressure from going sky high when I hand my key to the man at the service desk.

It is possible to return the driver's seat to your setting after a mechanic works on your car. I have short legs so I can't touch the pedals unless my car seat is pulled forward. It's difficult to pull the seat forward using just my sound hand because the runners bind if I don't apply a perfectly symmetrical force. It's easier to control the sliding motion so the seat will catch exactly where I want it *if* I pull on the steering wheel with my hemiplegic hand as well as my sound hand. To keep from using trial-and-error to reposition the seat, I keep a ruler in my glove compartment that lines up with a permanent mark I've made on the shift lever cover. When I think my seat is positioned correctly, I place the ruler flush with the front edge of my seat and check to make sure the end of the ruler is touching the pen mark. I go to a car wash that lets the driver stay in the car. I usually keep cars for ten years, so I learned the hard way that it's a bummer if you let a car body get rusty before you are ready to trade it in. I don't know how I will swing the cost of another car so I'm taking care of this one.

Was the money I spent for driver training well spent? My answer is a resounding "Yes." Driving makes meeting people for a social event a breeze. It makes shopping faster and easier. If a storm is coming, I can run out to pick up one item and be home in twenty minutes. I bought a four-door car so I can load packages on the back seat of the driver's side. I keep a small **folding cart** in my trunk to transport my purchases to my front door. I still use Paratransit services when there is really bad weather or my car is in the shop, but driving has been a boost to my self-confidence. I feel smug when I walk up to my car with my cane, unlock the door, and get in. I am slow on my feet these days, but I am as fast and safe as any sane, able-bodied person when I drive a car. The cost of gas and car insurance takes a big slice out of my limited budget so I have to do without other luxuries, like cable TV. People who live on fixed incomes can't have everything they want, but I am ecstatic about being able to drive a car.

Showering While I'm On the Road Again

Before you travel, you need to be sure you can **shower** at your destination. I don't want to give up going on vacation or visiting friends and family because I don't have access to a handicapped bathroom. I shower away from home by taking a light, folding shower bench made by Invacare. I found one at a local medical supply store that was listed in the yellow pages. This folding bench is light enough to be opened and closed one-handed, which means it is not heavy enough to stay still if you don't sit down gently. This <u>folding bench is not safe if</u> you need a grab bar for substantial support during a tub transfer or you are particularly heavy.

Since I don't have a shower hose to aim the water, I position the bench slightly out of the stream of water and lean into the stream to rinse. The best way to position the bench varies from bathroom to bathroom. If the showerhead looks like it is pointed down at the floor, I sit facing the faucets. If the showerhead looks like it is pointed at the back wall, I sit facing the back wall with my back close to the faucets. Sitting close to the faucets lets me twist around to control the temperature settings. If I see that the bench is not positioned correctly after I sit down and turn on the water, I turn off the water for safety before I reposition the bench. Whether I am facing forwards or backwards, I soap up and always lean *forward* to rinse. However, it's not safe to lean too far forward so I bring a large plastic cup to dump water on areas that are hard to rinse. I practiced using this shower bench in my guest bathroom at home before I left so I was confident it would work.

Next you need to make sure you can **transport** your shower equipment. Only a really large suitcase will accommodate the width of a folding shower bench, but it fits into a nylon garment bag. After I fold the nylon garment bag in half, I slip the nylon handles over the long handle of a rolling suitcase so the nylon bag hangs down over the front of the rolling suitcase. Then I place a smaller bag on top of the rolling suitcase. This smaller bag has a flap that slips over the handle of the rolling suitcase that keeps it in place. I can push this combination of rolling luggage a short distance, like from the curb to the front desk of a hotel, but I can't handle it at the airport. Someone suggested wrapping the bench in bubble-wrap to protect it from baggage handlers, but I've only used it when I've driven to visit so I haven't tried the bubble-wrap yet. If special shower equipment and procedures made it possible to go to the Caribbean or your grandson's house, would you give them a try?

A Plane Sounds Better than an MRI

The roar of jet engines and the excitement of flying is heaven compared to the deafening clang and anxiety I associate with an MRI. Of course, if flying makes you a nervous wreck, feel free to skip this section. If walking long distances is tiring, reserve a **wheelchair** when you call your airline or make an on-line reservation. *Do not call the* *airport.* I reserve an aisle seat because it is easier to get in and out of. Airline seats are crammed so close to each other that inching sideways like a crab to get to the middle or window seat is a challenge even for able-bodied people.

After calling my local airport, I learned that bus drivers who pick up passengers in remote parking lots aren't allowed to get out of their vehicle to put luggage on the bus. I will never be able to lift my luggage up those bus stairs, so a friend drives me to the airport. When my friend drops me off at curbside, the skycap checks in my luggage and puts it on the luggage belt for me. He calls for the wheelchair and prints out my boarding pass. The going rate for tipping is one to two dollars per bag. I didn't use skycaps when I was healthy, but it is a great way to reduce stress at the airport.

The airline employee who pushes me in the wheelchair has always arrived promptly and helped me through security. A great part of this deal is that airlines don't want their employees standing in line for hours, so you go to the head of the security line. I would be willing to present a copy of my letter from Social Security Disability when able-bodied people feel provoked by the increasing numbers of disabled seniors and abuse this wheelchair privilege. Once I get to the security gate, the steel shank in my orthopedic **shoes** causes some excitement because it sets off the alarms. The security staff in each airport handles this problem differently, but they have always been helpful and polite. Some airports have a screened-off area where I can sit down to take off one shoe so they can run it through the X-ray machine. Once I get through security, the employee assigned to me delivers me to the departure gate.

One problem I didn't anticipate when flying alone was how I would maneuver during the long wait at the departure gate. Waiting passengers have to go to the bathroom, handle a carry-on bag you can't leave unattended, and purchase food because airlines don't serve meals anymore. On my first flight, the employee left the wheelchair so I could push it around with my carry-on bag, coat, and purse resting on the seat. It is not safe for you to push a wheelchair around by walking if you cannot use both hands to steer the wheelchair around a crowded airport environment. On my second flight, the employee had to take the wheelchair with her. I was lucky because it turns out that every airline keeps a wheelchair at every gate that is folded up and kept out of sight.

Getting on the airplane offers some challenges. The first time I got on a plane, I suddenly became aware of the two-inch lip at the front door of the plane that I had to step over. I never paid attention to this obstacle before my stroke. I can walk down the aisle to my seat, but airlines have narrow **wheelchairs** to transport people who can't walk. These narrow wheelchairs don't have armrests. When you raise the armrest of an aisle seat out of the way, you can get to your seat by sliding your bottom over and then moving your legs over instead of standing up and walking sideways.

I made the mistake of letting the stewardess standing at the door stow my carry-on bag at the front of the plane. She told me to wait for the steward who sat in the last row of the airplane to get my bag down for me when I got off. My friends thought I hadn't arrived because the steward and I were the last two people off the plane. On the return flight, I checked my carry-on bag to avoid this lengthy delay.

Going to the **toilet** is easy for me because I can walk down the aisle while gently resting my sound hand on the tops of the seats. I could use my **cane**, but if there is sudden turbulence I don't want to smack someone with my cane as I reach out for support. I'd rather have my sound hand free to hug the top of someone's seat than to fall into a stranger's lap. Unfortunately, I can't tell you what people do about getting to the bathroom if they are wheelchair bound, need a walker, or require a lot of physical assistance to walk.

An airplane bathroom is tiny, which can be a blessing. The wall is close enough to lean your forearm against to steady yourself if turbulence hits while you are sitting on the toilet and to help you stand up when you are finished. I don't know what people do if they need a grab bar to stand up. The edge of the sink is close enough to push off of, but I have never tried this because all the airplane bathrooms I've been in have had the sink on my hemiplegic side. I don't trust my hemiplegic arm to support me in a moving vehicle.

When your plane lands, an airline employee will meet you at the door of the plane with a wheelchair. He or she takes you to baggage claim or an intermediate drop-off site where other employees with electric carts stop to pick up anyone who is sitting in the waiting area. You have to know your flight number so the employee knows which baggage claim area to head for. Retrieving my luggage is easy because the friend or family member who meets me lifts my luggage off the conveyer belt and carries it.

Flying is relatively easy for people with physical disabilities because airlines have had to comply with the American with Disabilities Act (ADA) for years. It may be new to you, but the employees know what to do. Just remember that you have to do some extra planning before you go to the airport.

Returning to Work

I can't return to my job as a full-time professor of occupational therapy. The obvious reason is my paralysis. I no longer have enough active movement in my right arm and leg to demonstrate evaluation procedures and treatment techniques for the physically disabled. The invisible deficits of poor balance, the inability to multitask while standing, and low endurance also interfere with my ability to work.

Poor **balance** interferes with my ability to teach labs. I can walk in a straight line in an unobstructed area, but if I stop, turn my head, and attend to someone unexpectedly I lose my balance and stumble. Students often ask questions while they are standing behind me in a lab and I would genuinely be afraid of falling if I turned to answer them. Lab space is inadequate where I taught, so extra chairs, therapy equipment, and students' belongings were often in the way as I walked around to different groups. I used to trip over these obstacles before I had a stroke. I can't imagine how I would safely navigate this obstacle course now. Does your job require good balance to maneuver around obstacles?

My inability to **multitask** while standing interferes with my ability to teach large lecture classes. I need to stand to see all the students, not just the first two rows. I need to move around to engage many students in the discussion and see if a student in the back looks puzzled but is too shy to ask a question. I need to see if students are fidgeting to help me decide if it's time to give them a break. I need to repeatedly get up to run videos and slides. Running videotapes and slides to a specific spot to answer a student's question is hard to delegate. I need to stand up and turn 180 degrees to write on the blackboard. I can't lecture, do all this moving around, and keep my balance too. How much multitasking does your job require? Are you allowed to work uninterrupted in a quiet area?

Low **endurance** contributes to my inability to work full-time. I don't have the stamina to commute 105 miles a day and work six days a week including evenings, which is what teachers do. I can compensate for paralysis by using one-handed procedures, but I can't rest in the middle of a lecture. I perform best if I go to bed at 10:00 p.m. and get up at 7:00 a.m. Just when I think I've beat the limitation of low endurance, I push myself too hard and end up having to go to bed early or sleep until noon the next day. If you go back to work, think about starting part-time to give your body time to adjust to the workload. Even sitting for hours can be tiring at first.

I enrolled in the national Ticket to Work program when I agreed to mentor a small group of students taking a research course that required discussion around a table. The Ticket to Work program allowed me to stay on disability while I worked part-time to learn how hard it would be for me to work again. If I earned more than $900 a month in 2007, the government would send my disability check but count that month as part of my nine-month return-to-work trial period. If the months aren't consecutive, like a teacher who doesn't teach in the summer, the trial period ends when you work for nine months over five years.

I decided not to continue teaching occupational therapy part-time. There were two deal breakers in addition to my right-sided paralysis, limited endurance, poor balance, and inability to multitask while standing. First, I can't drive safely in rush-hour traffic on the interstate so the department's entire schedule would have to revolve around giving me a mid-day class time. This is a big accommodation for the faculty to make on a permanent basis. The two other OT programs in my state are even farther from my home so I would never be able to teach without using an interstate. Second, I discovered that I need a wife. Returning to work would be more doable if someone had my dinner ready when I got home and had my laundry done so I had clean clothes to wear the next day. However, my part-time work

131

experience gave me the confidence to become an ESL tutor in my county.

I'm glad the Ticket to Work program allowed me to explore work-related problems while Social Security disability checks gave me a reliable source of income. If you want to return to work after you have a stroke, go to www.ssa.gov/work/aboutticket. Click on Service Provider Information to find the agency that administers the Ticket to Work program in your state. The ssa.gov website will tell you how much you can earn each month without jeopardizing your disability status. Type "substantial gainful activity" in the website's search window.

You will probably have different deficits than I do, but describing my experience may make you more aware of the obvious and hidden challenges you have to take into consideration. An OT can help you evaluate your ability to go back to work. He or she will be familiar with the American with Disabilities Act (ADA) and can recommend reasonable accommodations you can request from your employer. If you qualify for vocational training, I recommend that you take advantage of it before you go back to work.

The Bottom Line

This chapter illustrates why having a home health aide visit a few hours a week isn't enough to keep stroke survivors in their homes. Even if you are independent in self-care and do some homecare, you may still end up in an institution if you can't handle advanced ADLs in the community.

Therapists don't think about training stroke survivors to participate in community activities because they treat clients in the hospital, when they are homebound, or in outpatient clinics. It's a mistake to assume that stroke survivors don't need to do ADLs in the community because "the family can handle that." My doctor wants to see me every four months, nine prescriptions run out at different times and have quadrupled my trips to the pharmacy, grocery shopping never ends, and shopping for clothes can be like going to war. Asking one person to run all the errands and take a stroke survivor to every appointment and activity is expecting too much because our needs go beyond the ordinary.

You will probably need a variety of strategies to succeed. If you have a healthy spouse or adult children who live nearby, you may be able to delegate some ADLs in the community, like shopping. Primary caregivers need to think ahead. Your support system is going to disappear if you keep saying "thanks, I can do that" to people who **volunteer** when a stroke survivor first comes home from the hospital. One of the kindest things people can do to help a stroke survivor is to run an errand for the caregiver. Ask a friend or neighbor to take a package to the post office or pick up stamps. Finally, stroke survivors need to think about regaining independence in some community-based ADLs to take pressure off of the people who care for them. For example, taking the Paratransit bus to some daytime activities can be a big help. Stroke survivors and their families have to think about these mundane tasks because not being able to manage ADLs in the community may be the tipping point that forces you to leave your home.

CHAPTER 7

PAIN CAN RUIN EVERYTHING

There is a hitch to my glowing story of recovery. Pain can ruin everything. It is discouraging when pain forces you to stop using a body part that has been injured. Forced rest causes you to lose some of the gains you've worked so hard for. Eliminating pain isn't always possible, but managing it usually is. This chapter talks about getting pain under control without using drugs. Pain makes you feel helpless, so knowing you are in control is half the battle. The other half of the battle is using techniques that are specific to the different causes of pain. Here are some problems frequently associated with stroke that can be painful.

A Subluxed Shoulder Really Hurts

A subluxed shoulder is painful because the upper arm bone (humerus) has slipped partially or completely out of the shoulder socket. Subluxation is rated by how many fingers you can fit in the space created by this joint separation. I had a one-finger subluxation so the hospital staff gave me a small lap tray that slid over the armrest of my wheelchair to keep my hemiplegic arm supported. The staff had to take off this lap tray every time I got out of the wheelchair. I made sure they put it back on because I knew that if my subluxed shoulder wasn't supported, the nerves in my arm could be damaged from being overstretched. The lap tray also gave me a place to rest my hand palm up. This palm-up **hand position** helps roll the upper arm bone outwards, which puts tension on the glenohumeral ligament. When this ligament is taut, it helps the muscles hold the shoulder in the socket where it belongs.

The lap tray didn't support my shoulder when I walked, did my self-care, and sat on a mat table to do exercises. My shoulder ached constantly during these times until my OT bound it up with Kinesio Tape. This tape is stretchy so it creates a great deal of tension without cutting off circulation when applied properly. My shoulder felt better as soon as David got all the strips of tape on my shoulder. I wore this special tape twenty-four hours a day, even in the shower. It eventually came loose and had to be replaced every third day.

Even with the Kinesio Tape on my shoulder, it hurt when I leaned forward to reach for something because my limp arm flopped forward. That jolt felt like someone was punching me hard on a sore, achy shoulder. Initially I tucked my hemiplegic hand in a "crease" I created by raising my sound thigh to trap my hemiplegic arm close to my stomach. Later when I regained voluntary shoulder and elbow flexion, I was able to hold my bent arm close to my chest. Today I can hold my extended arm by my side when I lean over.

I'm proud to say that I beat shoulder subluxation three times. I worked very hard at it because it really hurt. The solutions I've described work best when shoulder subluxation first appears. To discover if you have a subluxed shoulder, use your sound hand to feel your shoulder joint. You shouldn't be able to feel any space because the shoulder joint should be very tight. If your shoulder is subluxed, do everything that your therapist recommends.

Vigilance Fixes a Swollen Hand

I was very aggressive about treating my swollen hand because trapped fluid presses on nerves, which is painful. I didn't have a badly swollen hand, but I've treated many people with strokes who did. I've never forgotten the client who came to therapy with a swollen hand and was in so much pain he said, "You're not going to touch my hand, are you?" I didn't want my swollen hand to hurt that much.

Elevating your arm is the best way to bring down the swelling in your hemiplegic hand because water runs downhill. When my hand was swollen, I religiously put my forearm on the lap tray of my wheelchair when I was in the hospital and on the table when I ate at home. My mother taught me it wasn't polite to rest my arm on the table, but I think she would understand if she were still alive. I put my hand on a pillow at night even though I knew it wouldn't stay there all night. If you have a swollen hand, follow through on any recommendations your OT gives you.

A Cold Foot Can Ruin Your Sleep

An unexpected source of discomfort was my cold hemiplegic foot. When winter arrives, my foot is ice cold by the time I go to bed. I didn't know a cold foot could keep me awake for hours after I crawl under the covers. When I put a heating pad over it, it initially takes an hour for my foot to warm up. To save electricity, I put the heating pad on a timer like the kind that turns house lights on and off when you go on vacation. After a month or so, it takes only fifteen minutes for my foot to warm up. What a relief. If an ice-cold foot is ruining your sleep, see if this helps.

Do Shoulder Range of Motion Lying Down

Why should you range your shoulder? Therapists are serious about shoulder range of motion because they've seen clients who don't move their shoulder get shoulder-hand syndrome. This is a very painful condition in which the arm and hand become stiff and the lightest touch is painful. The only treatment is to range the shoulder. Clients cry non-stop through this procedure. They also cry every time their hemiplegic arm is lifted during dressing and bathing. You don't want to get shoulder-hand syndrome.

When I was a therapist, I taught clients to do shoulder range of motion while they were sitting. I thought this was a good idea because I never sat down and tried to lift my client's hemiplegic arm over my own head. There is a good reason why therapists stand and use two hands to pick up your hemiplegic arm. A hemiplegic arm is heavy, either because it is limp or because it is tight and resists movement.

It's easier to range your shoulder while lying on your back on the bed. First, gravity helps your arm go where you want it to go. Lie on your back and lift your hemiplegic arm up towards the ceiling. Once you get beyond 90 degrees, gravity pulls your arm down so it rests next to your head. Second, instead of straining to hold your arm overhead, your sound arm relaxes because the bed supports the weight of your hemiplegic arm. When the sound arm relaxes, the hemiplegic arm relaxes and is easier to stretch. Third, the bed cons your hemiplegic arm into thinking it is time to rest (yeah!), so you are more likely to prolong stretching rather than rush through it. My hemiplegic shoulder is tense at first when I get my arm next to my head. I have to wait several seconds until my muscles relax, my arm sinks into the bed, and I achieve maximum range.

However, there is a precaution when you range your shoulder. It is convenient to lift your hemiplegic arm by digging your fingers into your forearm muscles. Every time you dig your fingers into muscles you stimulate them, just as your leg kicks when a doctor taps your knee with a mallet. I avoid digging my fingers into my forearm muscles because I don't want to stimulate muscles that produce the painfully flexed wrists and fisted hands I've seen in other stroke survivors. Instead, lift your hemiplegic arm by grabbing the long bones on either side of your forearm. Place your sound thumb parallel to the bone on the thumb side of your forearm while your fingers contact the bone on the little finger side of your forearm. Do shoulder range of motion the safe way by grabbing your forearm correctly.

How Do You Relax Tight, Painful Muscles?

One of the most difficult things stroke survivors have to learn is to relax muscles that are tight and painful. It isn't a matter of trying harder. When it comes to relaxing tight muscles, less is more. Here are some tricks that make me more comfortable when I stretch. Remember, the true goal of stretching is to relax tight muscles rather than do a large number of repetitions.

Stretching is like coaxing a puppy. If you try to train a puppy to sit or lie down by pushing forcefully on its rump, the puppy stiffens up and fights you. The same thing happens when you forcefully stretch a tight, painful muscle. Instead, move your limb only as far as the muscle is willing to go. When you feel resistance, stop and maintain moderate rather than maximal pressure until you feel the muscle relax a little. Wait. Relaxation can take up to a minute when you first start stretching. When the muscle relaxes and you start stretching again, move slowly. Move so slowly that someone has to watch closely to even see the movement. If you enjoy moving quickly as I do, you will know you are moving slowly when it is as irritating as fingernails-on-the-blackboard. Repeat what I call "stop-wait-stretch again" until the muscle won't relax anymore. Stretching feels good when you take advantage of the slack that a muscle gives you when it relaxes a little. Your muscles will look forward to stretching this way. The advantage of doing your own stretching is that you can feel when muscles relax and are ready to let your limb go farther in the range.

However, it is difficult to be patient when stretching a tightly fisted hand. I had the patience *not to* force a client's hemiplegic hand open when I was a therapist, but got angry when my own hand would not open. Here are some steps that helped me relax my hand.

Stretching the Hemiplegic Hand

1. With the hemiplegic hand palm-down, *slowly* bend your wrist down towards the forearm as far as it will comfortably go. Bending the wrist downwards forces the hand to open, if only partially. When you feel resistance, repeat "stop-wait-stretch again" until the wrist won't relax anymore.
2. Keep the wrist flexed and *slowly* straighten the thumb. The thumb is the powerhouse of the hand so stretching it first makes the other fingers relax. It's ideal if you keep your thumb open as you do step
3. I keep my thumb open by trapping it against the base of my sound thumb when my sound hand grabs my hemiplegic fingers in Step 3. A caregiver may need to hold your thumb open by grabbing your thumb with their whole hand (no pinching with bony fingertips).
   Keep the thumb straight and *slowly* straighten the fingers. When you feel resistance, repeat "stop-wait-stretch again" until the fingers won't relax anymore.
4. Keep the fingers as straight as you can and *slowly* push your hand back like cops do when they raise their hand to stop traffic. You may get frustrated if you can't get your wrist all the way back. <u>Warning: Do not cheat by</u> bending your fingers backwards at the first knuckle. This overstretches small muscles on either side of the first knuckle that you need to control finger movement. Keep your palm and the first knuckle of each finger in a straight line. When you feel resistance, repeat "stop-wait-stretch again" until the wrist won't relax anymore.

Some days your hand may be so tight that you can't open it at all. When this happens, put your hemiplegic hand on your lap. Use your sound hand to *slowly* roll your forearm back and forth so your hand rolls from palm up to palm down and back. This may relax your hand enough so you can go back and at least do Steps 1-3. If you do Steps 1-3, they will help you open your hand to wash it.

I wear a hand splint at night to help maintain the gains I achieve with stretching. I am on my third splint because the first two eventually broke in half at the wrist. This tells me the high muscle tone in my wrist muscles is bending the splint when I sleep. I gave up on heat-molded plastic splints and am currently using a SaeboStretch splint. This splint is designed to bend and spring back. You can learn more about this splint at www.saeboflex.com.

Stretching can be boring unless . . . Stretching is boring even for a therapist who understands how important it is. Rather than ignore the stretches I am supposed to do, I spread them out. I divide them into short segments based on the time of day and the task I'm doing. I love doing some stretches in the morning while I'm still under the bedcovers. It's easier to stretch when my muscles are toasty warm. Stretching is also a great excuse for staying in bed another ten minutes. It's like having your mother tell you to get up and then forgetting about you. I feel like I'm getting away with something.

I pair some stretches with specific tasks. For example, I stretch my shoulder just before I put on my shirt. This stretch is easy to fit into my daily routine because I need to lie down on the bed and rest for a minute after taking my shower before getting dressed anyway. I prefer to stretch my hemiplegic hand when I'm watching TV. Being distracted by the TV helps me be patient if my hand tightens up when I try to open it. For me, setting aside a big block of time in a schedule that changes from day to day feels like a burden. I prefer to stretch by finding a few minutes here and there throughout the day.

These are a just a few examples of how to make stretching easier to do. See if my strategies trigger ideas that work for you. Therapist's instructions are not set in stone. It's better to be creative than to give up stretching altogether.

Straining undoes your hard work. It is counterproductive to stretch and then strain excessively during other activities. You are probably straining too much if a movement makes you hold your breath, fist your hemiplegic hand, or curl your hemiplegic toes. When I feel signs of straining, I make my exercise program easier that day. The first thing I do is to rest between contractions. This strategy is amazingly successful at getting a tight muscle to relax. However, this doesn't always work so my second strategy is to cut down the amount of resistance I'm using. I reduce the number of pounds I am lifting or switch to lighter objects. My last strategy for cutting down on straining during exercises is to come back later that day when I am more relaxed. See if you can finds ways to keep straining to a minimum when you are doing activities.

I have the hardest time practicing what I preach about stretching when I'm doing ADLs I want to finish. Here are three strategies that can help me relax during a functional activity. First, I take a deep breath and wait for a few seconds. For example, if I am having trouble getting my hemiplegic heel down into my shoe, it helps to stop and take a deep breath and wait a few seconds to give my toes a chance to relax and stop pointing. The second strategy that helps me when I tense up during an ADL is doing something to distract myself. When I'm trying to hook my bra and the hooks keep slipping off the eyelets instead of catching, I stop and briefly listen to the radio in my bedroom that I turn on while getting ready in the morning. Third, changing my **position** may reduce straining. When I'm struggling while trying to pull a pullover top down in back, standing up helps. I don't know why. Maybe the effect is just psychological, but I don't care because it works. See if you can find procedures that keep straining to a minimum when you are doing ADLs.

A fourth strategy that helps tight muscles stay relaxed during ADLs is **good positioning**. Poor positioning takes a while to make muscles strain, but the negative effect is real. Sitting in the wheelchair while waiting to be transported to therapy taught me that good positioning takes only seconds and really pays off. I made sure an aide put the lap tray on my wheelchair so it would support my subluxed shoulder and make it less painful later on. Even now that I can walk, I practice good positioning in sitting. For example, I keep my hemiplegic hand in a good position while working for hours at the computer. I put a *cone-shaped* spray bottle in my hand with my little finger at the wide end. The wide bottom makes it easy to rest the bottle on a surface. To keep the bottle in my hand, I took the top off the spray bottle and attached a vertical strip of self-adhesive **Velcro** that I slip my fingers under. I scotch-taped a small piece of **Dycem** next to the Velcro strip to rest my thumb on to keep it straight. What activities do you do regularly that put your body in a good or bad position for long periods of time? Do your positioning choices tighten or relax your muscles?

The Bottom Line

Pain can ruin everything. I can honestly say I have consistently used the techniques in this chapter to reduce pain and to prevent it from coming back. However, there isn't one solution. Reducing pain requires solutions that are matched to the specific cause of the pain.

CHAPTER 8

RECOVERY OF A PERSON

A stroke paralyzes an arm and leg that belongs to a person. During my early recovery, I focused on learning to control my body at the expense of everything else. As physical issues receded, I was able to concentrate more on my recovery as a person. This chapter talks about depression, regaining a social life, and how a stroke changed my outlook on life. The healing process is slow, but I eventually found a whole new life worth living.

Choosing to Live

It takes more than cheery self-talk to deal with the **despair** that is a natural response to a stroke. The first month after my stroke I prayed every night that I would die. When I woke up each morning to find I was still alive, I started to think about suicide. Without my asking, the rehabilitation hospital sent a psychologist to talk to me in my room. Doug's first visit came about three weeks after my stroke. We never talked about suicide, but I could see in his eyes that he knew I was thinking about it. I couldn't see the point of living if I wasn't useful. Helping others is a big part of what motivated me to become a therapist. Doug kept asking me about what I wanted to do after I got well. I thought he was crazy, but he came by once a week and kept talking to me in a gentle, patient way about my plans for the future. It took a year before I fully understood and appreciated how Doug had influenced my recovery. He had planted a seed of hope without my being aware of it.

Doing meaningful activities again was a major factor in my choosing to live. The recreational therapist lent me a book easel so I could read, which I love. I was able to maneuver my wheelchair independently one month after my stroke so I wasn't stuck in my room all the time. By the second month, I was able to roll my wheelchair outside to sit in the warm spring air. I'm an outdoor person and don't think I can be in a bad mood when I'm outside. Then I was over-the-moon about being able to shave my legs. Six weeks of hair growth made me feel like "Gorilla Woman." The day that my OT helped me shave my legs, everyone I ran into heard about it. My friend Arlene suggested I keep notes so I could write a book about my stroke experience. Karen and Lynne, two coworkers from the university where I taught, visited me. Suddenly I was talking about how the admission of the new class was going. Each of these meaningful activities gave me a break from obsessing about being dependent for the rest of my life.

The loving kindness of people was another factor in my emotional recovery. One day a friend visited and kissed my cheek. My therapists had to touch me, but Pattie didn't. Suddenly, I could feel the encouragement that everyone was giving me. My brother Mark flew in from Illinois to see me. His visit meant a lot to me in ways I cannot explain. The avalanche of love coming toward me suddenly felt real.

I don't know when I stopped thinking about suicide, but I do remember telling myself that I should wait to see how things turn out before I make any drastic decisions. Somewhere along the line, I got caught up in life again.

Regaining a Social Life

My recovery as a person includes regaining my social skills. Loved ones can be hurt if they take the initial selfishness of a stroke survivor personally. I hope my story helps family and friends understand why social skills may be lost at first and gives them hope that they can return.

Being self-absorbed conflicts with an adult's self-image. When you are in the hospital, the nurses want you to tell them quickly what you want. This kind of terse communication about what you need doesn't go over well in the real world. When I went to live at my friend's house, I didn't have the social grace one expects of a friend. Family and friends expect you to say "hello" and "how are you?" at the beginning of a conversation, but I would ask for something I wanted first. Although I remembered to say "thank you," there was no genuine feeling behind it at first. Suddenly switching to walking everywhere at home was exhausting. For weeks I had to focus on what my hemiplegic leg was doing. I fell if I let my concentration lapse even for an instant. I was physically and mentally exhausted every day for two months after I left the hospital. There is a crushing level of fatigue that doesn't leave any energy for social interaction.

My experience with a dog illustrates how fatigue can interfere with social relationships. Kodiak used to go nuts every time he saw me. His owner knew how much we cared for each other so she walked him to Arlene's house to see me. He was old and going downhill, but lived only two short blocks away. When he arrived, he glanced at me and lay down. He stared straight ahead and acted as though I didn't exist when I petted him. Walking those two short blocks took every ounce of energy Kodiak had. Seeing Kodiak focus so intently on just breathing made me realize that social skills are a luxury you can't always afford.

I was despondent because I knew how self-absorbed I was. I had regained control of my body but had lost the caring person I used to be. If I had known that social grace would slowly return as fatigue lifted, I wouldn't have felt as much despair. I was eventually able to say "thank you" with genuine emotion when I was free from the tyranny of paying constant attention to controlling my body. If being self-absorbed sounds familiar, try not to be as hard on yourself as I was. See if your social skills return when you are not so tired.

Talking to strangers. When I got to Arlene's house, I practiced my social skills by saying hello to strangers. She lives in the center of a small town where people speak to each other on the street. When I could walk outside without constantly looking down at the ground, I started to think about the people around me. People who make eye contact with a handicapped person are taking a risk because they don't know what to expect. I decided to set people at ease by being the first one to say hello. Once I spoke to them, people usually looked me in the eye, smiled, and said hello back.

Making Paratransit reservations, doctor and therapy appointments, and calling utility companies also gave me practice talking to people. Those phone conversations made me realize that I got lucky when it came to dealing with strangers. Instead of having a spouse speak for me, I developed the confidence to talk to people instead of becoming socially withdrawn. Look for opportunities to talk to people. Just saying hello, making eye contact, and smiling are a good way to start.

I stumbled on a gracious way to respond when strangers try to help me when I don't need it. Kindness can quickly turn to embarrassment if people feel rebuffed. When I was in rehab, I heard another client say "thank you for offering." I tried using this phrase and it works. When I thank strangers for offering to help, 99% of people have smiled. People feel good when I tell them their offer makes me feel safe. I never know when I might need help and appreciate knowing that strangers are watching out for me.

Show me where the fun is. It took about six months after my stroke before I had the energy to ask where the fun is. Fortunately, a shock I had before my stroke gave me the incentive to reach out to other women. An elderly woman and I had talked at church for four months before I realized that most of the people she was talking about were buried in the cemetery behind the church. I didn't want to end up lonely in my old age. There are a lot of women who are divorced or widowed, so we might as well as get together.

There are several safe ways to socialize as a single older woman. I joined a book discussion group at a bookstore in a small town rather than go to one at Barnes & Noble. A few people in the group went out for a drink afterwards. After a year this book club disbanded, but some of these women formed a group that meets for breakfast once a week. I've joined a local writing group that is sponsored by the International Women's Writing Guild. You'd be amazed by the number of women who have personal stories that are burning to be written. I've joined a new church that offers a wide variety of activities that provide the opportunity to socialize, such as dinners, discussion groups, and volunteering. The library system in my county offers free meeting space to clubs, like a genealogy group. There are safe ways to meet people who share your interests that aren't as expensive as golf or going on a cruise.

I'm looking forward to turning sixty-five when I won't be the only "baby" at my senior center. The senior center in my town offers a wide array of activities. It offers physical activities, like bocce ball, aerobics, yoga, and line dancing. It offers sedentary activities, like low-cost hot lunches, a movie night, a video-lending library, and board games like checkers and Scrabble. It brings in attorneys who provide free legal aid, trained **volunteers** who give free advice about Medicare, and staff from a local hospital who conduct health fairs and free health screenings. It offers artistic activities, like painting, a choral group, a band, a poetry club, and trips to theatrical performances in New York. The center arranges trips to Atlantic City and vacation spots, like Colonial Williamsburg. Senior centers realize that today's elderly have a wide range of interests.

Of course, small towns can't afford to provide all of these services, but adjacent towns could join together to pool their resources the way hospitals share expensive MRI equipment. This proposal won't work in the sparsely populated western states where towns are hours apart, but it has potential elsewhere in the United States. Local bureaucrats may resist giving up exclusive control of senior services, but some unruly baby boomers need to use their protest skills to push towns to provide the services we want. Baby boomers are going to stay active and senior centers can help. Before you wrinkle your nose at the idea of going to your senior center, call or go on-line to get a list of activities.

While having fun is one of my major life goals, recovery as a person includes deeper issues. Conversations with friends and family helped me reassess four ways I look at the world: (1) my need for perfection, (2) my approach to stress management, (3) my tendency to get depressed, and (4) my mistaking want versus need. Just listening to myself talk and getting their feedback about what I had said was helpful.

My Perfectionism Comes Back to Bite Me

The old me. I don't know why doing a task perfectly makes me so happy. I've enjoyed spending half an hour using Q-tips to make an old toaster spotless. I felt a sense of pride that I don't have a grungy-looking toaster just because I've had a stroke. It annoys me if even one ice cube gets stuck in the tray. My four siblings and I probably fought

146

over having to share the ice cubes when we were kids. Throwing away one ice cube after it melts in the tray really bugs me, so I always spend the extra time to repeatedly whack the tray until the last ice cube comes out. However, being a perfectionist is not good for my blood pressure.

The revised me. A funny thing happened while I was learning to make a bed one-handed. At first it looked as though a child had made the bed. I eventually learned to make it perfectly, but it took so many trips around the bed that it was exhausting. One morning I stopped when there were still a few wrinkles in the top cover and the pillow was sitting on top of the bedspread instead of tucked under it. I paused and thought, "This is how a man might make a bed." I had to laugh because I realized that men are on to something good. It takes a lot of time and energy to do something perfectly. Making a bed perfectly uses energy I can save for something that is fun or important. I could have another stroke tomorrow and I'm not going to regret that my bed isn't made perfectly.

A friend who has taken advanced business seminars said I needed to use the 80 per cent rule. This rule states that some tasks have to be done perfectly while other tasks have to be only 80 per cent perfect. The rule says that achieving the last 20 per cent to make something perfect takes 80 per cent of your resources. A savvy business manager chooses which jobs deserve the extra resources to make them perfect. Businesses teach their managers to use the 80 per cent rule so I've taken it to heart.

It wasn't easy for a perfectionist like me to use the 80 per cent rule at first, but when a task takes lots of time or effort I stop and give it a chance. Here is one example. I found an easier way to tie my shoelaces. I used to meticulously tie them super-tight, going back over every lace twice to make sure there wasn't any slack. Now I tie my shoes quickly and retighten the laces only if needed. I get my shoelaces super tight on the days I go shopping. Other days I just get them pretty tight, which is okay for walking around the house. Leaning down in sitting for a long time to tie my shoes increases my blood pressure, so applying the 80 per cent rule to this task has done wonders for my health.

My perfectionism is still here, but it is more selective. I'm not expending lots of energy doing everything perfectly. Now I aim for perfection when it pleases me, like getting all the ice cubes out of the tray, or because it's necessary, like making my shoelaces really tight when I walk in the community. My perfectionism still takes over at times, but having a stroke has transformed my life. If perfectionism is making your life stressful, consider the 80 per cent rule.

Stress Management Gets Out of the Back Seat

The old me. It's amazing how much energy I've wasted feeling guilty about what I didn't get done. I've spent time revising to-do lists and looking for logical rationales for what I should do next. Logic is a puny weapon against a formidable enemy like guilt. It feels like I've wasted entire years that I wish I could get back.

The revised me. I discovered that starting with a task I feel strongly about often gets me unstuck. The day still ends with some tasks undone, but I accomplish more if I get started and move from one task to the next than I do if I spend time feeling guilty about what isn't getting done. Here is a procedure I stumbled on that gets me going when I'm stressed out.

I call this procedure "reverse-meditation." I lie down on top of the bedcovers with my clothes on. I don't have to worry about falling asleep because I've never been able to nap in the middle of the day. Instead of trying to empty my mind as traditional meditation recommends, I let my thoughts ramble. In about ten minutes, these fleeting impressions become a single train-of-thought that won't go away. Suddenly, I'll realize that I'm thinking about a task that has been bugging me without my being aware of it. Putting a load of clothes in the washing machine is a relief after realizing I've been watching the clean clothes dwindle every time I reach into a drawer. Instead of adding one more task to a long to-do list, this sudden insight energizes me and makes me jump up from the bed because it's a task I really want to do. Who knew it was possible to decide what to do next without any angst? I get to rest for twenty minutes and sort out my priorities without getting a knot in my stomach. Amazing!

I also do a traditional form of meditation to feel less stressed. I sit comfortably with my feet flat on the floor and pay attention to my breathing. It takes about ten minutes for my breathing to slow down and become deeper. Staring at a candle with my hands clasped in front of my belly makes me feel less fidgety. This simple meditation can lower my blood pressure by twenty points. I bought a blood pressure device made by La Crosse Technology that slips on the wrist. It self-inflates with the help of two AAA batteries. It cost $50 but is very accurate. I took it to my doctor's office and he got almost the same reading with a conventional blood pressure cuff. I've known for a long time that meditation is good for my health, but I never set aside the time to do it. Meditation isn't just for Tibetan monks anymore.

Retiring doesn't mean you don't have stress in your life. Meditation and "reverse meditation" are just two examples of how to reduce stress. Explore ways of reducing stress that you can relate to. Stress management has to get out of the back seat after you have a stroke.

Being Depressed for Hours Instead of Months

The old me wasn't too bad. I've always had the tendency to get **depressed**. One habit that helped me before my stroke was writing in a gratitude journal. When my sadness is unrelenting, my gratitude journal shows me that I'm not paying attention to the wonderful things that happen around me every day. For example, when I drove to work a group of birds sat on a particular lamppost over the on-ramp to the interstate I took every day. It amazed me that they always sat an equal distance apart. Some looked down at me while I looked up at them. What were they thinking? We were a part of each other's morning routine and it made me smile *if* I remembered to look up. The other day I saw a grandmother wheel a shopping cart into the grocery store with her grandson sitting in the mock automobile section of the cart. He had both hands on the wheel and a serious look on his face. When his grandmother turned the shopping cart, he conscientiously turned the steering wheel in perfect unison. When I saw this, I smiled.

Letting moments of pleasure pass by without noticing them is a symptom of something more serious. It means I'm worrying about the future or ruminating about the past instead of paying attention to what is happening right now. Not being fully present had become such an ingrained habit that even major delights flew by me after a brief "that's nice" reaction. Writing in a gratitude journal taught me where happiness comes from. For me, happiness comes from paying attention to the wonderful things I have in my life right now.

Writing in my gratitude journal goes in cycles. When I get back in the habit of appreciating joyful moments as they are actually happening, I stop writing about them. In time, this awareness fades and I start to feel depressed again. Antidepressants take six weeks to be effective and have negative side effects. Once I start writing in my gratitude journal again, it takes about two weeks before I live in the present and feel joy. Life is good when you're not waiting for the best part to begin.

The revised me is even better. After my stroke, I stumbled on a second procedure that improves my mood. I call it making a want-to-do list. This list doesn't contain any "shoulds" that I've generated with a logical analysis of what needs to be done. My want-to-do list contains items I'll enjoy that day, even returning a library book so I don't have to pay a late fee. I write my list on a Post-it while eating breakfast. I throw the Post-it out at the end of the day and don't look at it to see what I didn't do. I even refuse to feel guilty on the days I skip making this list. A want-to-do list is an amazing antidote for depression because it puts me in touch with my *feelings*. I enjoy life and accomplish more when I am aware of my preferences instead of making a long list of things I *think* I should do. Starting with a task that makes me feel good gives me momentum that jumpstarts the rest of my day. I still get depressed, but it's for hours or days instead of weeks or months.

Going to a stroke support group also gave me a more positive outlook. It helped me realize that losing the use of one hand isn't the worst thing that can happen to you. I met a woman who hasn't been able to say more than three-word phrases for sixteen years due to a language deficit called aphasia. Another woman had a stroke in her thirties and lost custody of her three children when her husband divorced her. There is always someone worse off than you, which is perversely comforting.

Go on-line to find stroke support groups in your area. The American Stroke Association lists support groups in your area in the "Life After Stroke" section (www.strokeassociation.org). The National Stroke Association lists support groups in your area in the "Stroke Survivors" section (www.stroke.org). Some universities run stroke support groups. The speech therapy department where I used to teach supervises graduate students who run support groups for stroke survivors with language problems. Support groups usually have a general meeting and then break into separate meetings for stroke survivors and caregivers.

You might consider talking to your doctor about taking medication. A doctor started me on an antidepressant in the Intensive Care Unit as a preventative measure. I took an antidepressant for a year without any side affects. I don't know if the antidepressant helped, but I certainly don't think it hurt.

Depression is a natural reaction to having a stroke, but that doesn't mean you have to accept unrelenting sadness for the rest of your life. If hopelessness has impaired your quality of life, I hope my examples inspire you to find ways to deal with depression.

Love and Lust

Family can be a great source of emotional support. How a stroke survivor re-enters the emotional life of a family is complex. I am not qualified to talk about the deep issues that require couples therapy, but I do have a few thoughts to share with you.

Partners. When I think about still being married and having to cook, clean, and do laundry for two people, my eyeballs roll back in my head. It's all I can do to take care of myself. I have two words for couples who want to have a great relationship and keep the house looking the way it used to: Maid Pro. I'm not sure that it makes a difference which spouse had the stroke. Able-bodied partners are going to be worn down. They have to do the chores their partner used to do, continue to do the jobs they were doing before the stroke, and care for the stroke survivor. As someone who is doing the work of a husband and a wife as well as taking care of myself after a stroke, I can tell you that this is an outrageous amount of work for one person.

Stroke survivors can't afford to ignore how their stroke affects the relationship with their partner. If certain tasks are a constant source of friction or resentment, get creative rather than fight. One woman I met had a husband who wasn't interested in cooking before or after her stroke. Her solution was to eat out once a week, order in pizza once a week, have her adult son cook once a week, and make light dinner meals on the other nights. Consider dipping into your savings to pay for maid or yard service if chores are a constant source of stress. Paying for homecare services costs less than a nursing home or assisted care. The difference is hundreds versus thousands of dollars each year.

If you can't afford to pay for outside help, consider asking your family for help. Paying for lawn care is one way a son or daughter who lives 2,000 miles away can help. Caring for parents who have broken up after one parent has a stroke puts even more stress on your family. Consider swallowing your pride and asking for help with tasks that are eating away at your relationship. It's easier to prevent the damage that constant friction or resentment causes than to undo it.

While a long-term relationship would be a great source of support for me, I am concerned about the energy it will take to find, build, and maintain a new relationship. Just watching couples flirt or stare into each other's eyes makes me tired. I foresee my fatigue undermining any relationship. Stroke survivors have to be realistic about what they promise to do to support a relationship.

While I'm discussing relationships, it's a good time to talk about the emotional lability that often accompanies stroke. Emotional lability is an excessive or inappropriate emotional response to a situation. The emotion may start out as appropriate, like crying when something is sad or giggling when you are nervous, but the response can be prolonged and exaggerated. These emotional outbursts create stress in a relationship. Anyone who has had hiccups has some idea of how emotional lability works. It's a neural circuit that is stuck in the "on" position. I've kept crying after I'm no longer upset. Emotional lability usually recedes as time passes, but it still ambushes me at highly emotional events, like a funeral.

Friends have stopped my emotional lability by putting an arm around me. The sooner they do it, the sooner I quiet down. Therapists who work with hyperactive children know that constant pressure calms the nervous system. I don't know if my friends' approach works because it calms an area of the brain called the Reticular Activating Formation or because I believe it will work. I am just glad it works. A toddler who has a temper tantrum gets to take a nap afterwards and sleep like the dead as only a young child can. As an adult, I get to beat myself up about making a scene. Ask your partner if he or she has discovered something that helps him or her calm down when emotional lability strikes.

Sex. I haven't had the good luck to have sex since my stroke, but there is one thing I know for sure. Film directors choreograph lovemaking scenes and then make actors rehearse them until they are perfect. You don't hear actors in movies saying, "Honey, I would prefer it if you would . . ." Filmmakers don't create role models for real people who have to negotiate if they want to have enjoyable sex.

While I don't have solutions, I do have concerns about sex. My hemiplegic foot feels like it's burning when I touch it. Will a partner touching my foot create an unbearable distraction? Abnormal sensation is common after a stroke. Lying on my hemiplegic side is uncomfortable because this shoulder is deteriorating. Is there a **position** that is uncomfortable for you? I am concerned about the timing of sex relative to when I take a water pill (diuretic) that helps control my blood pressure. I experience frequency and urgency for several hours after I take this water pill. Frequency means I have to go to the bathroom several times. Urgency means sometimes I leak urine if I don't get to the bathroom soon after I feel the urge to go. I can wear a panty liner during the day, but can I prevent incontinence during sex?

153

Abnormal sensations, painful positions, and medications are a few examples of issues that can affect your sex life after a stroke.

A Stroke Teaches You Want versus Need

I slowly began to differentiate between what I want and what I need. I want a heavier car that has a nice ride. I need a lighter car that gets good gas mileage so I can afford to pull it away from the curb. I want a car with cruise control, electric windows, a CD player, and a sunroof. I need a car I can afford. A car significantly reduces the time I spend running errands so I can have a social life and volunteer as an ESL tutor. I need to feel useful and have fun because they make surviving a stroke worthwhile.

When I moved out of my three-bedroom house, I had to give away about a third of what I own. This taught me more about need versus want. It was a pleasure to see friends and acquaintances beam when I gave them an object they really treasured. I gave my mother's wooden recorder to a teenager who had been performing with a plastic recorder. When she came to thank me, she was so happy that tears were rolling down her cheeks. That beautiful musical instrument had been sitting in my closet for years. After two years of giving things away, I was amazed at how many possessions I had hoarded without using them. I am at the point in my life where I have accumulated so much stuff that I have to throw something away in order to find a place to put a new purchase. Arlene, who owned a gift shop, taught me that you don't have to own something to appreciate it.

The liberating experience of giving away things I no longer use helped me adjust to living on a fixed income. After being a good consumer all my life, I was surprised to learn that the impulse to buy often passes. The object isn't always that appealing a day or two later. If I wait, sometimes I remember that I already own something that does the same thing. Knowing the difference between want and need makes it easier to decide what to buy. I'm not sad that I can't impulsively buy a product that sits in a closet as long as I can buy things that are really important to me. I'd have a lot more money in my retirement account if I had learned the difference between want and need before I had a stroke.

However, a fixed income does limit my social activities. My friends are in their forties, fifties, and early sixties when adults have more money. Now that I'm on disability I can't afford to go to expensive restaurants and performances. I have to say no to some invitations. This means the next time I get together with friends I listen in silence so they don't have to explain the events they are discussing that occurred while I was missing in action. I had fun with cash-poor friends in college, but it's hard to socialize when there is a wide range of incomes in a group. Maybe there won't be as big a financial gap when my friends retire. I need social interaction more than I need to buy what advertisers try to convince me to want.

The Big Question I Asked Myself

I've never asked myself, "Why me?" As a therapist, I've seen a lot of bad things happen to a lot of nice people. The big question for me was, "Why did I survive?" At first, I avoided asking this question by focusing on concrete things. It was easier to learn how to open a can of soda one-handed than to ask why I'm still here. I finally thought about the big picture when two lifelong friends who live hundreds of miles apart asked me the same question. Anne and Janet asked me, "Have you worked as hard as you have ever worked in your life to get back into your old ruts?" When I answered this question, I was surprised by what I learned about myself.

If my stroke had happened ten years earlier, I would have been devastated. When I was forty-eight, a lot of my self-worth was invested in being a teacher. Yet after being a therapist for six years and a teacher for eighteen years, I was ready for a change. I wasn't passionate about work any more. I had been asking myself what kind of work I should do next, but I didn't want to let go of the comfort of a familiar routine. I procrastinated until a bomb went off under me. After my stroke, I didn't have a choice about accepting change. I could have another stroke tomorrow so I'm in a hurry to do what I want right now. A stroke is unbelievably liberating because there isn't any time left to say, "I'll be happy when I have . . ."

When I let go of my identity as a therapist and a teacher, an amazing thing happened. The first project that found me was writing this book. It has been years since I've felt driven to write, since I've felt that a book had to be written and I was the perfect instrument. I've rushed to the computer so I wouldn't forget a great idea I just had. Ideas woke me up in the middle of the night. I didn't have peace unless I worked on it. This book wouldn't have been possible without the help of my friend Mirah, who took the photographs, and my friend Janet, who edited it and gave me encouragement when I needed it most.

My second project found me after I started outpatient therapy. My hemiplegic hand was making progress, but I couldn't prove it. I still couldn't pass tests that place a premium on speed, like placing small pegs in a pegboard as quickly as possible. When my hemiplegic hand became my assistive hand, I started writing down the tasks it helped me perform. Those notes turned into the Test of Early Bilateral Hand Use (TEBHU). In 2006, I field-tested the TEBHU on stroke survivors at a rehabilitation hospital. In 2007, graduate students in the OT program where I used to teach helped me field-test the TEBHU at another hospital. These two projects gave me a sense of purpose and dumped three years of work in my lap. Two more projects are on the horizon.

Having a stroke has changed my definition of purpose. I used to define purpose as a concrete goal I wanted to achieve. I think this point of view gave me tunnel vision. I let deadlines, which come regularly for a teacher, push my relationships to the back burner. "I'll talk to Sue tomorrow," I said to myself. I used to listen to people with the logical part of my brain. Now I take the time to listen to people with my heart. If I ask people how they are and really listen or share a funny story or smile and say hello, it's a good day. I see now that if I don't slow down and take the time to care for people in what seems like small, insignificant ways, my big accomplishments leave me feeling empty. I still set concrete goals and want to achieve them, but I've learned to take the time to connect with people in a genuine way.

Paradoxically, by really listening to what people are saying, I've learned to take things less personally. I've learned that a majority of people's thoughts have nothing to do with me. If someone is having a bad day, their being nasty usually doesn't have anything to do with me. Knowing this often takes away my anger about how that person has treated me or the anxiety I used to feel when I couldn't fix a problem. As the oldest daughter who was responsible for younger siblings, not feeling I have to make everything okay is huge! Of course, not taking things personally is easier to do with strangers than with family, but I'm learning to listen more to the people I love as well. One of the most important things we can do for someone is be a witness to what really happens to that person. This added layer of meaning makes life sweeter and broadens my understanding of purpose.

My stroke experience has changed my sense of self in the world. I used to feel that my being here on Earth wasn't particularly important. I used to feel like an interchangeable cog – a useful cog, but a replaceable one. If I weren't here, other people would do what I do. For the first time in my life, I truly believe that each person brings a unique set of talents to a task that can't be duplicated. I've been given a second chance and don't want to waste it. I want to do everything I can with the gifts and time I've been given and I want to enjoy doing it. I've stopped asking why I'm still here.

References

deMello, A. (1990). *Awareness*. New York: Doubleday.

Tolle, E. (1999). *The Power of Now*. Novato, CA: New World Library.

Appendix A

Assisted Living

Assisted living (AL) provides an apartment, three meals a day served in a communal dining room, and various forms of assistance for seniors who can no longer live at home. At a minimum, an AL apartment must include one unfurnished room, a bathroom, and a kitchenette. AL facilities typically offer group transportation to locations like the mall.

You can find AL facilities on-line, but beware. Websites like "momsplace" sound friendly, but remember that many listings are posted by for-profit corporations. In New Jersey, AL facilities are licensed by the state. The New Jersey Department of Health and Senior Services website posts deficiencies and complaints found at the last two state inspections. Log on to your state's website to see what you can find out about assisted living.

When I visit an AL facility, I don't want to be swayed by the lovely pictures on the walls and the friendly staff who take me on a tour. Some concerns are obvious, like whether the facility is clean and smells nice, but living with a stroke has made me a more discerning consumer. Learning about these two facilities showed me that I am concerned about (1) location, (2) prerequisite skills, (3) cost, (4) space constraints, and (5) the loss of personal freedom.

The following discussion is general because the specific information I received when I contacted two AL facilities is confidential. I don't know how representative these two facilities are so this appendix is an example of the information-gathering process rather than a survey.

Location may influence your decision. If you have a lot of choices, proximity to other resources may help you narrow the field. The obvious concern is how far away the facility is from your family. Being close to lifelong friends or a familiar church congregation can be equally important. Do you have a medical condition that requires frequent doctors' visits or hospitalization? Will you have to travel to receive therapy services? How far is the AL facility from these medical services? If you are still active, proximity to a senior center or college may be a consideration. Activity programs in some assisted living facilities can look remarkably like a nursing home's. Daily Bingo may not be your cup of tea. Senior centers and local colleges offer a wider range of activities than a single AL facility can provide. Paratransit services that take you to a nearby college or senior center can expand your options when you are in assisted living.

Prerequisite skills may limit your choices. Even wealthy people can't get around the fact that AL facilities don't take everyone. There are prerequisite skills that (1) can prevent you from getting into an AL facility and (2) allow a facility to force you to leave. Facilities that take seniors with Alzheimer's disease expect to deal with many self-care issues. Facilities that admit seniors who are frail or physically disabled may require you to have more self-care skills than an Alzheimer's unit. For example, what will happen if you become incontinent or can no longer feed yourself? You will eat three meals a day in a communal dining room, so you cannot neglect self-care. Do you need assistance with self-care tasks? Does the facility reserve the right to be the sole decider of how much care you need or will they consider input from other professionals, such as your doctor?

Can a facility accommodate someone with a stroke? I need adapted equipment to be independent in bathing. Will the facility let someone replace the regular showerhead with my long hand-held shower hose? Will I be allowed to put my shower chair in the tub? Is the grab bar for the shower and the toilet on my sound side? I currently walk with a cane, but may need a wheelchair at a later date. Do the apartments have wheelchair-width doors *inside* the apartment, like the bathroom door? A minimum of thirty-two inches wide is required and thirty-six inches is preferred if you have to turn a corner to get a wheelchair into a room. What accommodations do you need to ask for?

Cost may limit your choices. What is the monthly fee for different kinds of AL units? An AL unit can be a studio, one-bedroom, or two-bedroom apartment. How much has the monthly fee gone up over the past five years? An AL facility near my home has raised its monthly rent for a studio apartment $125 per month for each of the last four years. If I want to prepare breakfast in my room, do you offer a limited contract that only covers two meals a day? How much is the admissions processing fee? Does an occupational therapist evaluate your independence in ADL and a physical therapist evaluate your functional mobility? If you need help with self-care, how much does this assistance cost? If you need assistance in assisted-living, that costs extra. How often is assistance with self-care provided (e.g., two baths per week)? If I want self-care done more often, how much extra does it cost? Are housekeeping and laundry services included in the monthly fee or do they cost extra? Does the laundry service include both linen and my clothes? How often is laundry and house cleaning done? What activities does the facility charge extra for, like the beauty shop? How much does cable TV cost per month? If I go on Medicaid after I am admitted, will I be forced to leave?

How a facility charges for services like the ones listed above will determine your real cost. Before you decide what you can afford, don't forget that you have to pay for medicine, health insurance, the clothes on your back, telephone service, haircuts, toilet paper, and other expendables. And don't add up your monthly costs until you have read about space constraints.

Space constraints may limit your choices. The "one unfurnished room" in an AL apartment can be a combined bedroom, living room, and dining room. One 12-foot x 13-foot room I looked at had room for only a pull-out sleeper sofa, a nightstand, a small table, a small desk, and an upholstered chair. You can have a separate bedroom, but it will cost you more.

Space can be restricted in less obvious ways. An apartment may have only one closet. The mementoes you've accumulated over the years will not have a home. Where will you keep clothes and bed linen for all four seasons? Is there extra storage on site and does it cost extra? A kitchenette may not have space for a refrigerator, so having a sink and microwave oven may not give you much freedom to eat what you want. Larger AL units have a full kitchen, but if you are paying for three meals a day, a full kitchen isn't saving you any money. There is no place to put a small stackable washer and dryer, so you have to pay for laundry service unless you have access to a laundry room. Ask to see what a furnished apartment looks like to help you visualize space constraints. Then revisit the price list to see what your monthly cost would be given the space constraints you've discovered.

Personal freedom may be restricted. Will you be allowed to take your medications without supervision so you are not tied to the facility? I take medication four times a day and don't want to be homebound so a nurse can hand me my pills. How much choice does the menu give me? How often does the menu change? One AL facility I visited checks on residents who don't show up for a meal. How often does the van make regular trips and where does it go? Will the van take you to places that other residents don't want to go, like a doctor's office? If you still drive, can you come and go at any hour, do you have to check in and out, and where will you park? Are visiting hours restricted? Are pets allowed? What is the appeals process if you are dissatisfied? If the facility says you can no longer stay there, how much time do you have to find an alternative living arrangement? These intangible concerns aren't obvious so keep your ears open for constraints on personal freedom when you take a tour.

The bottom line. I've created a list of questions about assisted living. Asking for an information packet and talking to a representative on the telephone will answer some of these questions. Other questions are easier to answer when you make an actual visit. I list prickly questions on the bottom of page two because I don't want these questions to set the tone at the start of my tour. Questions about location are on the last page because staff wouldn't be able to answer these questions. First impressions are also on the last page. I want to think about my visit for a while before I write down my general reaction to the facility.

The following list is just an example. I didn't include a question about pets because I don't have any. I urge you to make your own list. You wouldn't walk into a car dealership before you formed some idea of what you want, would you? A list helps me learn what I want to know when a salesman tries to divert my attention with glossy brochures or sell me features I can't afford.

References

Matthews, J. L. (2002). *Choosing the Right Long-Term* Care: Home care, Assisted Living, and Nursing Homes, Chapter 3. Berkeley, CA: NOLO Publishing.

Name of facility_____

Date of Visit_____ Phone number_____

Person I talked to_____

Accommodate my stroke

- Will you let me put my shower chair in the tub?
  Does the showerhead have a long hand-held shower hose?
- Is the grab bar for the toilet and tub on my sound side?

Cost

- What is the monthly fee for different units?
  How are the units different?
- Do you have a limited contract if I prepare breakfast in my room?
- How much is the admission processing fee?
  Will an OT and PT help decide how much care I need?
  If I need help with self-care, how much does it cost?
  How many times a week will I be helped (# of baths)?
- Housekeeping: What services are included in the monthly fee?
  How often is house cleaning done?
- Laundry: Is all personal laundry (e.g., clothes, bed linen, towels)
  included in the monthly fee?
  How often will my laundry be done?
  Will the staff make my bed with the clean linen?
  Will I have access to a laundry room?
- What does basic cable TV cost?

Space constraints

- What are the dimensions of the unfurnished room?
  (A 12' x 13' room may have room for only a sleeper sofa,
  nightstand, small table, desk, and an upholstered chair.)
- How many closets are there?
  Is there any extra storage on site and what does it cost?
- Does the kitchenette have room for a small refrigerator?
- I want to see a furnished apartment.

Personal freedom

- Will you allow me to take my medications without supervision?
- What happens when I don't show up for a meal?
- Where does your van go?
  How often does your van make regular trips?
  Will the van take me to places other residents don't want to go, like my doctor?
  Is there a distance limit (e.g., 10 mile radius)?
  How much does this personal transportation cost?
- I drive in good weather so where will I park my car?
  Can I come and go at any hour?
- Do I have to check in and out?
- Are visiting hours restricted?

Questions for the end of the tour

- Do residents with Alzheimer's share communal spaces I'll be using?
- What does the activity calendar look like for two different months?
  Which activities cost extra?
- What does the menu for two different months look like (i.e., how often does the menu change)?
- When I exhaust my personal assets and go on Medicaid, can I stay here?
- What is the appeals process if I'm dissatisfied?
  (Someone in risk management writes up an appeals process to limit the corporation's liability.)

Location

The facility is close to

_____ Family   _____ Doctors   _____ Senior center
_____ Friends   _____ Hospital   _____ College
_____ Church   _____ Therapists

First Impressions

- Physical appearance and cleanliness

- Staff demeanor

- Residents and activities I saw

- Tidbits I learned along the way

- Deal Breakers

Appendix B

Concierge Service Anyone?

"The assisted living communities had better take notice," said Joseph Coughlin, who is the director of an MIT think tank on aging (Basler, 2005). He is talking about consumer groups that have created local non-profit organizations to help seniors stay in their homes. Beacon Hill Village (BHV) in Boston is a famous example. BHV describes itself as a comprehensive concierge service for people who live in the Beacon Hill neighborhood and are fifty years of age or older.

BHV helps with odd jobs. Suzanne Stark found herself calling BHV when she couldn't get her cat in a carrier so she could take it to the vet. Services also include discounted fees for carefully vetted professionals such as house cleaners, plumbers, personal trainers, caterers, computer advisors, and 24-hour care nurses.

Free services include a weekly car ride to the grocery store or doctor-prescribed medical procedures, exercise classes, and monthly lectures. Services that keep residents connected to their neighbors are weekly lunches in a local restaurant and day trips to places like the Newport Jazz Festival. Since many elderly residents feel isolated, these social activities are an important way to maintain a sense of meaning and connection.

I've looked into independent living facilities. They offer more upscale amenities (e.g., golf) and less personal monitoring because they admit only older people who are independent in self-care. Currently there are fewer independent living facilities in comparison to the number of assisted living facilities. Some independent living units are part of a continuing care retirement community (CCRC) that also has assisted living and nursing home units. Because CCRCs promise to keep you until you die, they require a hefty entrance fee that can range from $50,000 to $300,000 (Matthews, 2002).

BHV membership costs $600 a year per person and $850 a year per couple in 2009. Discounted memberships are available for low-income residents. Unfortunately, only a few states have these kinds of "villages." To see if there is a village near you, go to www.beaconhillvillage.org and click on Other Villages. The founders of BHV have written a manual on how to create a village in your neighborhood. The manual costs $350 for non-profits and neighborhood groups. The fee includes advice from BHV and help with a business plan.

Right now it is getting harder to take care of my home and walk community distances. I feel like a tire with a slow leak. Joseph Coughlin is right. When I need help caring for my home and doing activities in the community, I would pay $600 per year to get some free services, help with hiring vetted outside vendors, and access to social events. A village like BHV sounds like a good intermediate strategy for staying in my home longer.

References

Basler, B., 2005. *Declaration of Independence*. Retrieved on March 25, 2009 from http://www.aarp.org/family/caregiving/articles.

Matthews, J. L. (2002). *Choosing the Right Long-Term* Care: Home care, Assisted Living, and Nursing Homes, *Chapter 3. Berkeley, CA: NOLO Publishing.*

Appendix C

Council on Independent Living

If I have to spend down my retirement plan and savings and qualify for Medicaid, I won't have many choices. If I live at an assisted-living facility for two years, I may be able to stay on as a Medicaid recipient after I've given them a big chunk of money as a private-pay resident. However, I will be tied to that one facility.

If I try to move to another facility after I am on Medicaid, I could end up in a nursing home. The Supreme Court ruled that putting disabled people who are on Medicaid into institutions when they can function in a community-based setting is a violation of the American Disabilities Act (Magasi & Hammel, 2009). Yet only four states spend more money on community-based long-term care than they do on nursing homes for Medicaid clients (Gold, 2007). The National Council on Independent Living (CIL) can help you stay in the least restrictive setting. Counselors at CIL centers know a great deal about services for the disabled in your area and can act as advocates if you need help procuring services. Go on-line to locate the CIL center that is closest to your home (www.ncil.org).

References

Magasi, S. & Hammel, J. (2009). Women with disabilities' experiences in long-term care: A case for social justice. *American Journal of Occupational Therapy, 63*(1), 35-45.

Gold, S. (2007). *FY 2006: Medicaid expenditures for institutions versus community-based services (Information Bulletin 216 8/07)*. Retrieved August 2007 from www.stevegoldada.com.

INDEX

These key words are **printed in bold** in the text.

backwards rule 59, 68, 89, 90, 99, 100, 116

balance affects ADLs 19, 24, 26, 27, 29, 37, 38, 62, 100, 103, 110, 113, 118, 130

canes
   maneuver with 22, 23, 47, 93 110, 116-118, 129
   retrieval of 20
   using different types 23

carts 27, 29, 48, 88, 93, 97, 100 113, 114, 116, 124, 126

depression 6, 142, 149

Dycem 60, 85, 89, 107, 109, 141

endurance 7, 30, 32, 33, 103, 104, 121, 131

fall prevention 13, 20, 22, 23, 28-30, 64, 65, 75, 84, 93, 103

hand
   range of motion 137-138
   recovery of 38
   strategies for early use 44-50
   swollen hand 135
   task modification for 51

memory aids 13, 16, 29, 85, 86, 87

multitasking 25, 27, 52, 53, 110, 130

non-slip shelf liner 43, 47, 51, 60 64, 86, 88

positioning 16, 58, 91, 134, 140, 153

shoes
   airport security 128
   donning 66
   inserts 24
   tying laces 69-75
   winter boots 77

showering
   handling clothes 20
   in the hospital 8
   preparing the bathroom 60
   procedures for 45, 47, 62
   walk to the bathroom 23
   while traveling 126

toilet
   at night 23, 38
   flushing 22
   handle underwear 19
   in a restaurant 109
   on an airplane 129
   sit down on 15
   tear toilet paper 45, 109

transport objects 23, 34, 84, 87 108, 127

Velcro 61, 66, 69, 75, 77, 78, 87, 141

volunteers 10, 81, 82, 103, 105, 114, 118, 133, 146

walkers 28, 34, 93, 118

wheelchairs
   maneuver 17, 84, 107, 118
   when you fly 127-129

About the Author

Dr. Rebecca Dutton is an occupational therapist (OT) who specialized in stroke rehabilitation. She is a stroke survivor who currently lives in her own home. She has a doctorate in Educational Psychology and has taught OT students at Louisiana State University, Temple University, and Kean University in New Jersey. She is the author of *Clinical Reasoning in Physical Disabilities*.